Guided Imagery for Healing Children and Teens

Wellness Through Visualization

Ellen Curran

BEYOND
WORDS
Publishing
I N C

Beyond Words Publishing, Inc.
20827 N.W. Cornell Road, Suite 500
Hillsboro, Oregon 97124-9808
503 531 8700
1 800 284 9673

Proofreaders: Janis Hunt Johnson and Carol Franks
Design: Principia Graphica
Managing editor: Julie Steigerwaldt
Composition: William H. Brunson Typography Services

Printed in the United States of America
Distributed to the book trade by Publishers Group West

Library of Congress Cataloging-in-Publication Data
Curran, Ellen.
    Guided imagery for healing children / Ellen Curran
        p. cm.
    Includes bibliographical references
    ISBN 1-58270-041-9 (pbk.)
    1. Fantasy-Therapeutic use.   2. Imagery (Psychology)-Therapeutic use.
  3. Imagery (Psychology) in children.   4. Child psychhotherapy.   I. Title.

RJ505.F34 C87   2001
618.92'89414—dc21

                                                                00-045493

The corporate mission of Beyond Words Publishing, Inc.:
Inspire to Integrity

Contents

The Trekking Dial
  Pegasus (Difficulty Breathing)
  The Oxygen Planet (Asthma Symptoms)
  In the Canopy (General)
  The Tapestry Shawl (Inner Strength)
  The Big White House (Stress/Burdens)

DEDICATED IN THE MEMORY OF MY MOTHER, MARGARET M. PETERSON.

AND A SPECIAL THANK-YOU TO MY WONDERFUL HUSBAND, MICHAEL, AND MY TWO EXTRAORDINARY DAUGHTERS, ALLISON AND ELIZABETH. THANK-YOU TO CHRISTINE ANDREWS WHO HELPED ME TO BEGIN TO WRITE. I DEEPLY APPRECIATE ALL THE KINDNESS AND SUPPORT FROM MY FRIENDS AND FAMILY—TOO NUMEROUS TO NAME THEM ALL—DURING THE WRITING OF THIS BOOK. SPECIAL THANKS TO MY YOGA TEACHER AND FRIEND, BEV ROSEN, MY LIFELONG FRIEND, LESLIE FULLER, MY TEACHERS IN IMAGERY AT BEYOND ORDINARY NURSING, SUSAN EZRA AND TERRY REED (AS WELL AS ALL MY CLASSMATES). AND I THANK ROSEMARY WRAY FOR HER GIFT AS AN EDITOR AND AUTHOR'S COACH.

Introduction

"Images, indeed all thoughts, are electrochemi-
cal events, which are intricately woven into
the fabric of the brain and body."

-*Jean Achterberg*

Healing imagery is a way to use one's imagination
in a focused way to help the mind and body to self-heal,
perform, and recuperate on both a physical and emotional level, by honoring oneself and helping the small
voice from within to be heard. The noise of our society
is deafening and has been found to be physically and
emotionally stressful, causing a myriad of illnesses for
both children and adults. This high-pressure environment equally affects children with chronic or acute disease and injury, making it more difficult to cope with
their symptoms and overall feelings of being unwell. To
learn a state of "quiet" enables children and teenagers to
connect with their self-healing abilities, to strengthen
their self-esteem, and to enjoy their own imaginations at
the same time.

Guided imagery for healing uses the quieted, focused
mind to enhance its effectiveness by making the child or
teen more open and sensitive to the unconscious mind.
This quiet, inactive use of imagery is a very empowering
experience, and it taps into the deeper levels of feelings,
making it possible for the inner self to "be heard" and,
therefore, to be healed.

What is imagery? Simply, imagery is thought. For example, as you drive to work in your car, you begin to imagine the workday ahead of you. You can actually see your workplace, with yourself and your co-workers in some activity together. You start to rehearse, in the car, what you might say to someone or what your actions will be in certain situations. You probably don't realize it, but you are also bringing in many other senses and feelings, besides just the visual, to this thinking or imaging. For example, the thought or image of a certain person at work can provoke a feeling of happiness, humor, anger, or fear. You feel these emotions, and in your mind's eye, you begin to respond to those feelings. In this process you elicit images from within (the mind) and interact with these images through the senses (the body). In essence, you are imaging all the time without realizing it, or perhaps you have called it "daydreaming"! Thus, imagery is a combination of natural mental processes, using a visual sense as well as other senses, like hearing, smell, and touch. Bodily functions that are believed to be inaccessible can be activated through imagery. A common example used to demonstrate this process is to picture a slice of lemon in your mouth; the "imagined" sour taste prompts you to salivate. This is an example of how the body listens to the mind. The imagined lemon and its sour taste are just thoughts, but they can produce a real bodily response. Our bodies react to the sensory images of the mind. The body does not know the difference between actual events and imagery (or thought). The practice of conscious, focused imaging can bring you to a deeper level of mind-body interaction, which in turn can produce wellness. This is the essence of imagery's power.

Imagery is designed to help those with both short- and long-term symptoms to better manage their conditions. I like to describe this technique as "self-directed biofeedback" that can enhance other medical treatments and be a part of the wellness plan.

Now picture how children process the world around them, how much of their everyday existence is experienced through the imagination. They live in a world of images, dreams, and fantasy. Children are intuitive, creative; they are naturally imaginative. This is why the technique of imaging for self-healing works so well with them. The imagery concept of an inner advisor or "helper" comes easily to a child, as does a secret, invisible friend.

But for today's children, there are challenges to the imagination. We must realize that they have grown up in the very sensorial world of TV, movies, video, and the Internet, being part of the most "plugged in" society of all time. Even small children are exposed to extraordinary visual effects of every shape, size, and sound. Movies like *Jurassic Park* and *Star Wars* brought dinosaurs back to life and hurled the audience through space. TV programs are more interactive and creative, stimulating children's minds as never before. Thousands of images flash before their eyes and across their minds in a matter of moments.

The children of the last few decades have an expectation for the incredible that we as children never had. Simplistic thought or fantasy can elude these children because they have been exposed to such overwhelming external stimulation. Thankfully, children are very flexible and may be ready for some true quiet in their lives, taking the time to tap into their personal fantasies and images. And, believe it or not, they are still attracted to the images of kings, queens, fairies, and goblins. Guided imagery jump-starts the imagination, making it fresh and original once again. Guided imagery for healing takes the essence of children's imagination to a deeper level, making them well!

There are many imagery techniques that can be learned to help you or a child. Whether for a simple or a complex situation, imagery can help you care for an ill or injured child. Imagery can be used to control pain, to increase coping skills, and to decrease many symptoms—especially pain. It can be used before and after surgery, for children receiving chemotherapy, and for those having to tolerate any difficult procedure. Because it is self-empowering, imagery can affect emotional issues. It helps children and teenagers with fear, stress, body image problems, and depression. For chronically ill children, whose body integrity is greatly affected, imagery can increase their positive feelings and honor of "self."

Sadly, there are not many resources to be found on this subject regarding children. There is a plethora of books, tapes, imagery therapists, and seminars for adults. There are some children's books using guided imagery for creativity and relaxation, but rarely a word is mentioned in terms of self-healing.

In this book, *Guided Imagery for Healing Children and Teens*, my hope is twofold: to tell of my daughter's journey from illness to wellness and to explain the powerful technique of imagery as part of a wellness plan. Parents, nurses, therapists, physicians, and any wellness practitioner will find *Guided Imagery for Healing Children and Teens* a moving story as well as an easy-to-use manual, which will open the door to a new and creative form of self-healing. I believe any parent can use this book in the home. It can also be a training manual for any caretaker, including the school nurse, home health worker, or the practitioner working with inpatients. It explains how imagery can be adopted as part of the intervention for uncomplicated symptoms such as toothache or itchiness, or even for severe and complex issues that arise from a diagnosis of cancer, asthma, or the need for an organ transplant. These more serious conditions can also entail difficult treatments and procedures that can be aided by imagery. Healing imagery gives children increased self-esteem because they can control, to a degree, some of the complicated feelings that accompany illness or injury. A sense of trust and personal power, as well as the formation of a unique bond of compassion with your child, can also be accomplished by using this technique.

As a guide, you help create a safe place for children to explore their conditions, their symptoms, and their feelings about them, and to recognize or discover their needs. You help them to respect their inner world, thereby allowing the quiet exploration of its truths and insights. This applies to any technique, whether using directed, "read" guided imagery or Interactive Guided Imagery^SM. You are not acting as an interpreter. They are having their own unique experience with imagery; they are becoming aware, getting their own answers, and beginning their own healing process.

The following is a personal experience I had when I was training in imagery. I hope it will help you understand your role as a guide for a child a bit better.

The Sistine Chapel: Part of my professional imagery training through the Academy of Guided Imagery (AGI) included an exercise on the purpose of guiding. The exercise, guided by Martin Rossman, M.D. (co-founder of AGI), was a way to get in touch with my personal feelings and beliefs as a guide and to give them an image, in other words, to manifest my thoughts through imagery.

After I did my relaxation exercise, quieting myself, I went to my "special place" and connected with that image of beauty, safety, and peace. When I say connected, I mean that I was able to "be there" with the sights, sounds, smells, and essence of my special place. I was then asked to recall a time, in detail, when I was guiding a patient in imagery. Listening to Dr. Rossman's gentle voice, I began to get in touch, as a guide, with the particular qualities and values I experience, which include creating health, helping others, and caring. Slowly, I began to see an image of the inside of the famous Sistine Chapel in Italy. My eyes became focused on Michaelangelo's *The Creation of Man*, zoning in on the outreached hands in that fresco. I saw myself standing amidst that magnificence, smelling the candles, hearing the prayers, and feeling the presence of a higher power. All my senses were at work. The feelings of beauty, spirituality, and strength I felt were extraordinary. I could see every detail of the painting and even imagined back in time watching the great painter, Michaelangelo himself. I was greatly aware that the fingers of the two hands in this painting were not touching, giving me the sense that again the power of imagery does not come directly from me, but from the patient. I became aware that I was just the guide but the guide, nevertheless, in an incredible journey.

To this day I still do this exercise. It has become an important part of my overall practice, both personal and professional. I feel it keeps me clear about my original reasons for incorporating imagery into my life and medical practice. It also keeps me humble and aware that it is not my process, but the child's.

This book is easy to read and understand. It begins with Allison's story, then moves into general information on imagery and mind-body medicine. It provides you with suggestions for beginning healing imagery with children or teenagers, including some ways to become comfortable with working with your child (patient). In preparation for your role as guide, there is a section for you as parent to experience imagery for yourself. This exercise produces a unique personal knowledge into imagery as well as insures a comfort level with it when you work with your child. You can audiotape the imagery in *Guided Imagery for Healing Children and Teens* and use it anywhere, anytime. Learning to accept and honor your child's needs and inner voice gives you a new, clearer point of view to perhaps an old and difficult situation, as with illness. This clarity enhances the parent-child team in many ways.

Guided Imagery for Healing Children and Teens is peppered with real case studies of my interactions with children and their families. In addition, there are readily available problem-solving strategies throughout the entire book. Also available to you are blank pages for note taking. While doing an imagery session, it is important to jot down bits of information that you want to remember, making personal notes or journaling about your feelings as a parent or caregiver. This documentation can be used for sharing important information between parents, with other family members, and with medical personnel. *Guided Imagery for Healing Children and Teens* explains guided imagery for several different symptoms, with scripted imageries that are easy to read to a child or teen with an illness or injury. It also contains a section with instructions on Interactive Guided

Imagery^{SM}, which is an in-depth technique of imagery where children interact with their own images. Finally, there is a chapter on creating your own imagery with your child, where your creative abilities will shine.

Once you and the child are "trained" in this imagery technique, it can be done anywhere, anytime. I have used it over the telephone with positive results! This technique works in stressful situations. For example, if your child requires stitches for a laceration repair, I have found—both in my nursing practice and as a parent—that if the parent stays calm and in control of the situation, and does a powerful, directed imagery with the child, it will help prevent an escalation of the stress and trauma for both the child and the parent.

Imagery allows you and your child to enter into the new experience of healing from within. It can be used for multiple symptoms and conditions. Imagery works well with small children, teenagers, and adults. No one is too young or too old to learn and benefit from the powerful technique of therapeutic imagery.

Interactive Guided Imagery is a service mark of The Academy of Guided Imagery, CA.

A Note to Parents

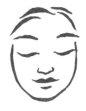

THROUGHOUT this book, you'll find an illustration corresponding to each guided imagery exercise. Please note that these illustrations are only brief hints at the imagery theme to spark the child's imagination. We have purposely chosen not to include elaborate drawings so that children and teens will not rely on the illustrations but will instead use their own fertile imaginations to create imagery unique to their symptoms and healing methods.

All of the imagery exercises can be used by both younger and older children, but the exercises in chapter 6 are more geared toward teens than the exercises in chapter 4. To help differentiate between the two, the word "teen" accompanies the exercises that were created with older children in mind.

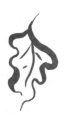

CHILD'S FACE: This icon signifies an individual case study

QUESTION MARK: This icon serves as a warning to problems you may encounter.

LEAF: This icon signifies general, helpful, interestin information.

One: *Allison's Story*

"IT IS ONLY WITH THE HEART THAT ONE CAN SEE
RIGHTLY; WHAT IS ESSENTIAL IS INVISIBLE TO
THE EYE."

-Antoine de Saint Exupery

ONE pediatrician called my two-year-old daughter Allison "the daycare baby" because she was always sick and I was a working mother. As a mother and a nurse, I felt that there was more to her clinical picture and that the physicians were missing something of importance. That day, I left the pediatrician's office vowing to find someone or some treatment that would help us.

Allison had two more years of continuous respiratory and viral illnesses. She had severe nasal congestion, cough, and recurring ear infections (which were affecting her hearing), always accompanied by high fevers. As our fear and worry escalated, we spent a great deal of time in many different physicians' offices for examinations and laboratory work. Unfortunately, despite these measures, we could get no firm answers about why she was sick all the time and required antibiotics on almost a continuous basis. Allison's fragile condition became more pronounced as she grew through her toddler years to pre-school age. Medications worked only for a short time or not at all.

Allison's overall poor physical condition was affecting her emotionally—making her tearful, shy, and fretful at three years old. At one point, the pediatrician advised that her adenoids should be removed. Out of sheer desperation, we allowed her to have this operation, in hopes that it would make her well. To our dismay, it did nothing to change her condition. Exasperated with her continuous illnesses and the ineffective surgical procedure, we insisted on further investigation by her new pediatrician. At four years old, Allison was diagnosed with profound, primary immune deficiency, meaning she was unable to mount any defense to infection. She had made no antibodies from her immunizations, and never would; there was no safety net. This was a very frightening revelation. With further extensive research, we found immune deficiency to be a murky diagnosis, with elusive treatment and an inadequate research program. And I vowed, as many other parents before me, "I will do anything I have to do to help my child." The initial plan of care was to place Allison on daily antibiotics, and if she "broke through" and became ill, a more potent antibiotic would be used.

At this point, I began to expand our avenues of treatment and implemented several dietary changes, homeopathic immunity boosters, and therapeutic touch. I also began using guided imagery techniques, to relax her when she was agitated, in pain, or having difficulty falling asleep. We limped along in this way for quite a while, dealt with the acute episodes of illness when they occurred, and tried our best to give the emotional support she needed, all the while worrying about the possibility of a catastrophic illness.

Despite our best efforts, Allison continued to deteriorate physically and emotionally. By the second grade, she was immature for her age and was having difficulties at school. She stopped functioning by 1 P.M. every day, displaying no stamina or tolerance to noise or schoolwork. She cried easily and was always at the school nurse's office. She experienced three episodes of pneumonia within a short time and missed many days from school (which affects her still, two grades later). This is when we realized that we had to take her to the next level of care and start intravenous gamma globulin infusions. This medication would give her the antibodies she needed to fight infection, at least temporarily. Synthesized antibodies would need to be infused every three weeks. This process required a six-hour infusion that usually included a post-transfusion reaction, such as vomiting, headache, and fever. And so another phase of this disease process was affecting both Allison and all of us, as a family.

Finding Imagery

"IF WE DID ALL THE THINGS WE ARE CAPABLE OF, WE WOULD LITERALLY ASTOUND OURSELVES."
-Thomas Edison

ALLISON'S RELAXATION RESPONSE was already in place from our previous imagery experiences. I believed that her imagery skills could be expanded so she could have a positive impact on her disease process and coping skills. I felt there was nothing to lose, since I held on to my parental vow.

We began our own special, guided imagery of the "Blue Whales" with her during her intravenous infusion. After the induction of a relaxed state, I asked her to imagine that powerful, Blue Whales were in every drop of intravenous fluid and that they were there specifically to make her feel better. They were hers and hers alone. They were there to help her understand her symptoms, fight off any bad cells, and help her recover and heal. Her response to and belief in this concept was automatic. She picked the name the "Frownies" for her particular "bad" cells and ran with it. The Blue Whales fought the Frownies along with her ill feelings—and it worked the first time we tried it. With help from her "new friends," the Blue Whales, she was also able to handle post-transfusion sickness by picturing them battling the Frownies inside her body.

I found that integrating the medical treatments with the self-empowering imagery process met nearly all of her needs, treating her as a whole person, and not just as symptoms related to a disease. More importantly, I gradually learned to let go of the controls, to make it her process, her healing, and her way. Letting go is a difficult but positive lesson for the parent of a sick child. Accepting her needs and perceptions enabled me to honor her as a person in her own right.

I was absolutely amazed at the progress Allison was making, both mentally and physically, and at the positive impact on our family as a whole. This progress prompted me to investigate further. I spent hours researching, trying to find out more about imagery and the essence of mind-body medicine.

Allison now feels special because of "her friends," the Blue Whales. Her belief in the Blue Whales and her trust that they will help her run deep. A wonderful example of this feeling occurred the day after her first intravenous treatment, when she was sent home ill from school. We had to stop by the side of the road, and I helped her as she vomited. Afterwards, with a ragged smile, she said, "Blue flowers will grow there now, Mum." Always believing in a happy ending. With the combination of a mind and body approach and Western medicine, Allison is now a healthier and happier child.

Recall

"MAKING THE SIMPLE COMPLICATED IS COMMON-PLACE; MAKING THE COMPLICATED SIMPLE, AWE-SOMELY SIMPLE, THAT'S CREATIVITY."
                                                    -Charles Mingus

AFTER WORKING with imagery for a short time, Allison brought her process one step further, describing to me how she called her Blue Whales by sounding a silent whistle when she felt sick or scared in school. The

Blue Whales would answer the whistle and come to her aid, comforting her and helping her to decrease her symptoms. Her body would have an automatic response, much like provoking the relaxation response. She could imagine her Blue Whales once again entering into her body to help her fight off the feelings that the Frownies brought. This recall process is quiet, private, and quick and can be done anywhere, anytime. The gift of "recall" gives children a way to bring back the healing imagery in times of need, when a parent or perhaps medications are not available to them. It is very empowering! This "recall" process also helped ground her feelings, which as I discovered later, was another very important aspect of any imagery experience. One of the most wonderful outcomes about this technique is that Allison created it herself, dramatically decreasing her feelings of helplessness.

Recall can also be linked to what is known as a "trigger" or "anchor." This is a simple mnemonic, like tying a piece of string around your finger to help you remember something, but taken one step further. I have known people who rub a ring on their hand, twist a piece of hair, or touch a stone in their pocket (anchor) to help them trigger relaxation and/or the recall process. Having a physical object or device that is integrated with a particular response or feeling can help you bring that wanted feeling or response back when you need to.

Such recall is another method or tool for children to help them focus on the process and to intervene for themselves. Keep in mind that occasionally it can be difficult for a child to activate the recall process without a parental prompt. At these times, the parent/child partnership is really evident. For example, when Allison is experiencing symptoms and is having a hard time doing her recall, I can help by saying in our secret code, "Why not try blowing your whistle?" She is then reminded or "triggered" to activate her recall and imagery process. It can be as simple as going into a relaxed state or reading imagery from this book. Whatever trigger or anchor your child chooses to use is okay, and it should be private. Our "secret code" has worked well in several public places and has helped to decrease any self-consciousness Allison may feel.

Surprisingly, as I went on to specialize in imagery as a nurse, I found that the Mind/Body Medical Institute, Division of Behavioral Medicine, Harvard University, has a technique called "minis" that is quite similar to Allison's recall process! "Minis" are a small version of the relaxation response. A "mini" is used during any part of the day to decrease stress. The act of taking a deep breath, releasing tension in the body, and using a focus word can aid in the management of stress.[1]

Here is Allison's Blue Whales imagery.
(Remember to always do some
sort of relaxation prior
to doing imagery.)

The Blue Whales

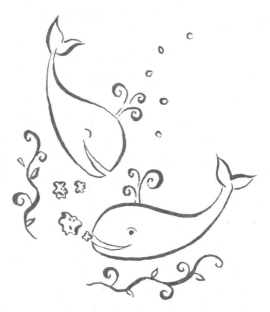

RELAX, shut your eyes, and breathe slowly and deeply. Quiet your whole body. Imagine the feeling of the flow of warm, blue-green seawater sweeping through your body. It feels like the whole world's oceans are within you, washing through you and calming you with every wave. Suddenly, you feel a tickling in your veins and you wonder, "What is that?" It comes again and again, and it feels good, so good that you start to giggle. Then deep inside you the answer comes. . . . "It is us, the Blue Whales." A million little whale voices answer you all at once. They actually sing their answer, and it sounds so beautiful and full of love. Your body is now their ocean, and they are playing and swimming in it. Imagine their shiny, blue brilliance and happy smiles. They are dazzling and magnificent. Even though they are tiny, they fill your body with their special healing power. They are here, in your body, to help you and make you feel well. Their power is becoming your power, and it is big, blue, and bold.

They have come to conquer the Frownies. The Frownies have been hard at work making mischief inside your body. They are the mean guys that live inside of you in small, round houses called cells. They love making you feel bad. The Frownies are not beautiful like your whales. They are dark, yucky gray, with big frowns on their faces. They want you to stay sick, or in pain, and to feel afraid. The Frownies do not like it when the Blue Whales come, because they know the Blue Whales can help you and make you feel well.

Now your Blue Whales will go after the Frownies with all their might and energy, and they will gobble up every one that they find. The Frownies run and hide when they see the Blue Whales, because the Frownies are cowards. But hiding does not help—because the Blue Whales are so smart and fast that they catch the

Frownies every time. The Blue Whales get big and fat and happy from eating all the Frownies. The Frownies may be mean and ugly to you, but they taste delicious to the Blue Whales.

You can feel them singing as they remove all the Frownies from your body. The Blue Whales shimmer throughout your body and are making you happy and strong again. You feel better, lighter, happier, and there is no more pain. The Blue Whales are your heroes. They love you with all their hearts and will always get rid of the Frownies for you ... any time ... any place.

Recall: Whenever the Frownies begin their mischief you can always call on your magical friends, the Blue Whales. Just shut your eyes, relax your body, and take slow, deep breaths. Now, blow a small secret whistle inside your body. Only you and the Blue Whales can hear it. When they hear your special whistle, the Blue Whales burst out of their hiding places in your body, where they have been sleeping in case you need them. They go right to work for you, chasing and eating the Frownies. They can help you get rid of your pain, your sickness, and any sadness you are feeling. Remember they are your special friends. Blow your whistle and let them come.

Two: About Guided Imagery

"WITH IMAGINATION ALL THINGS ARE POSSIBLE."

-Anonymous

GUIDED IMAGERY is used as an additional therapy in today's health care systems. It is used for a range of symptoms and situations, both minor and major, with extremely positive results. The following are some of the ways guided imagery has been used in many clinical settings and at home.

- Decreasing pain
- Relaxing and reducing stress
- Preparing for difficult procedures
- Giving the child or teenager a role
  in the wellness plan
- Increasing a child's coping skills
- Reducing anxiety and fear
- Helping in the preparation for surgery
- Boosting the immune response
- Improving sports performance
- Decreasing side effects from medications
- Helping to cope with chronic illness
- Enhancing body image
- Giving fresh insights/knowledge concerning
  a particular problem or symptom
- Empowering a child or teenager
- Enhancing speaking in public
- Intervening during a stressful or crisis situation
- Enhancing creativity and strengthening
  the imagination
- Lowering bloodpressure

(See p. 106 for the benefits of Interactive Guided Imagery.℠)

How to Believe in the Power of Imagery

"IMAGINATION IS ONLY INTELLIGENCE HAVING FUN."
–Albert Einstein

MANY TIMES I have seen blank faces when I speak about my practice with imagery as a wellness technique. When I go on to say that it is a powerful self-healing tool and part of the mind-body concept, I have observed many lost looks and occasional rolled eyes. But determined, I continue, detailing my twenty-four years of nursing experience, explaining the connection of the mind and body and my own daughter's healing process through imagery. At this point, I usually see faces change, and I get a glimmer of encouragement at this point. I keep talking. The key for my presentations and individual counseling is explaining the process well enough and interestingly enough to capture the most hardened skeptic, whether a child or parent. The minute I speak of my own experiences as the mother of a chronically ill child, an immediate connection is established. I tell of the worry and desperation I have felt as a parent, adding that the imagery process has been a success and a joyful experience.

One problem that must be dealt with is the reality that everybody worries. The concept of worry is an example of negative imagery, and it creeps up easily. Most of us can imagine events happening inside of our bodies. Many times the images come in the form of worry; perhaps we have a symptom that frightens us, like pain. We imagine something inside our bodies is going wrong. This usually makes the symptom worsen, which in turn causes a greater intensity of the symptom. What results is a powerful cycle of pain and anxiety. The good news is that, with imagery, we can imagine the good just as well. Due to lack of practice, we may not do it as well as we worry. If we can take that negative thought process and turn it into a positive thought process, we can overcome symptoms and promote self-healing.

I acknowledge the skeptics, as well as the people who are unaware of the technique of imagery, and their point of view. Many times what seems to be skepticism is really just a matter of having no experience with what imagery is and how it works.

I had display at a local Women's Health Fair and was doing short, individual imagery sessions for the general public. Outside my door was a sign saying "Guided Imagery." A typical response: a small, elderly lady asks me, "Can I take a look at your scanning machine? What are you scanning for?"

But forging ahead, I always tell my successful case stories about Allison and my clients, and then I go for the last point in my pitch, "a show of power." This is when I have my somewhat doubtful audience do a short, but powerful, imaging exercise. After relaxing with a deep breathing exercise (the launch pad of imagery), the parent and child are asked to imagine a "special place." A special place is a calm, beautiful, safe place in which they feel comfortable. Using sensory recruitment (as with the lemon slice), they can actually hear the wind, smell the grass, and sense the time of day in their special place, interacting with the sights, feelings, the "everything" of their place.

Once they imagine and reach their special place, it feels so real to them that, when the exercise is over, they have an obvious change in their attitude. This quick, concentrated imagery usually opens the lingering skeptics' hearts to the process, or at least it brings them a little closer to believing in the imagery process. Their ability "to image" is the first major step in believing in the process. Many people are inclined to think that they cannot image, but this belief is often false. Many are just too self-conscious, especially teenagers and adults. I have found that children rarely have this problem, but they may just be a little shy. The process of imagery quickly lets a child shed any shyness. Children can picture themselves easily. This is a very important gate to pass through for the seriously ill or chronically ill child or teen. I have witnessed both child and parents have a remarkable and deep experience on their very first imagery effort, thus firmly securing a positive attitude. The experience also illustrates very nicely that it is their power, not mine!

If the child responds positively to this experience, it is easy for parents to recognize this clear change in the child's attitude. Even if parents are doubtful before the exercise, I know they have accepted the child's decision to continue when they agree to put the child in my care, and I am honored when interaction occurs.

A reminder: Parents of sick children worldwide have promised, "We will do anything we have to do." Whether this promise is said when speaking to their own hearts, in the physician's office, or to each other, it is the driving force that they will live by while caring for a child with an illness or injury. Remember your promise if you get skeptical. Keep an open mind and, once again, trust in the process.

Frannie, a fourteen year old, had been complaining of a severe migraine headache for two weeks. She had missed school for several days and had been in bed taking multiple medications without relief. During her first visit, we did a short concentrated imagery. She was able to image her special place, in the forest, and relaxed somewhat. I asked her to imagine some kind of measurement device she could use to decrease her pain. She chose a wooden stick and started to make notches in the bark with a knife. Each notch represented a number. With each number she was able to decrease her pain. She rated her headache pain at ten (pain scale of one to ten, one being very minor and ten being very severe) and reported that she was able to decrease the headache to a three, notching her piece of wood each time. She was elated that the imagery worked and that she was able to do it herself. She continued using her pain control device at home and at school with success. Often, she was able to alleviate her symptoms, allowing her to remain in school.

Mind Body Medicine
(For the Right-Brained Person)

"THE BODY MIRRORS THE MIND AND SOUL AND IS
MUCH MORE ACCESSIBLE THAN EITHER. IF YOU CAN
BECOME PROFICIENT AT LISTENING TO THE BODY, YOU
WILL EVENTUALLY HEAR FROM THE WHOLE SELF."
        –On a blackboard at Harvard's Mind/Body Medical
                                              Institute

MIND-BODY MEDICINE focuses on the connections
between the mind and body and on how this connection
can directly affect health. We all have a capacity for self-
knowledge and self-healing, which unfortunately has
been diminished in our society over time. Emotional,
mental, social, and spiritual factors can influence how
we heal and how we stay well. What we need is to open
our minds and hearts to the concept of mind-body
awareness and to the techniques in which mind-body
medicine is grounded.

The cornerstone of the mind-body medical revolution is self-healing. But what is self-healing? It is a
difficult concept to grasp, especially for the Western
mind. Western medicine and science have evolved into
a rigid model, giving credence to pharmacology,
surgery, and the invention of "better" technology to
heal. Interestingly enough, it has been found over and
over that true healing comes from within. We are auto-
matically born with these profound powers to heal, but
we have rarely been taught how to use them appropri-

ately. These powers of self-healing are natural, easy to use, and free.

The most essential element of self-healing is simply believing and having faith in it. This faith gives us the strength to overcome the passive role of the patient, which in turn improves our natural, internal healing processes. Faith is strengthening. Another aspect that keeps the inner healer alive and well is self-care. When we incorporate a wellness plan in our everyday life, we can ensure good health and the power to self-heal. This wellness plan should encompass enhanced health practices such as yoga, imagery, nutrition, and relaxation. Self-healing also pivots off your lifestyle choices; the food you eat, the work you do, the exercise you perform, and the spiritual practices in your life all affect your capacity to heal. Taking these simple concepts and putting them into action, we can come to realize that health does not come from an outside source. It comes from within.

The patient population is changing and looking for new ways to control their own health care. There are many reasons why this has occurred; the American HMO crisis, dissatisfaction with conventional care, and increased access to the vast medical information on the Internet may be a few. But perhaps the real reason for this health care revolution is the realization that healing the person is more effective than treating the disease. Holistic medicine has become a ten-billion-dollar per year expenditure for American society and has entered the mainstream with a great surge, flooding into all aspects of care. Imagery is one of these holistic techniques. Using the imagery of the mind with some conscious effort can bring about physical changes in the body.

We are one unified organism. If we to pay too little attention to the mind, we lose a great deal of inner strength, something we naturally possess. Inner strength is the foundation upon which mind-body medicine practices have been built over the last two decades. This is not to say that imagery—or any other mind-body technique—is the only worthwhile form of care or that traditional medicine should be discarded. But with integration, the two philosophies will ensure a person-focused diagnosis and treatment plan. Medicine today is reaching back in time to the ancients for their expertise in treating a person as a whole. Integrating the latest scientific advances with the world's ancient healing systems will give people a way to stay well longer and preserve overall health for a lifetime. As the new millenium begins, we are in a tremendous medical revolution—the practice of medicine is being reinvented.

The concept of mind-body medicine has existed since the beginning of time but was lost to the Western world for many different reasons. A conflict between the patient and the scientist has existed for some time in the world of medicine. The patient needs to have hope, while the scientist insists on proof. Over the course of intellectual history, many philosophers, psychologists, and scientists debated the distinction between the mind and the body, from René Descartes to William James. Since the philosophical concept of dualism was accepted in the seventeenth century, the mind and the body have remained dissociated, especially in the field of medicine. The French mathematician and philosopher René Descartes suggested that the body did not need the mind to perform. His theory has been cited by today's scientists as an enormous impediment to the scientific exploration of brain function and has hampered Western medicine in the matters of integrating mind and body. At the turn of the nineteenth century, when there were immense advances in science, medicine, and industry, and the Western mind was focused on world expansion and discovery, the medical philosophy of the ancients, which was to consider the mind as well as the body as a whole, was rejected. In 1890, psychologist William James published the book *The Principles of Psychology*, in which he criticized any mind-body views of the day. At this pivotal point in Western medical though, there were many great advancements and discoveries, such as antibiotics, X-rays, and vaccination. Unlike the medicine of the past, which encompassed thoughts and feelings, these discoveries were supposedly concrete and scientific.

Mind-body medicine has evolved many times over since Dr. Herbert Benson, of the Harvard Medical School, gave the phrase prominence in the 1970s. Dr. Benson was attracted to the notion of a "scientific" Dalai Lama. He traveled to the Himalayan Mountains to study with Tibetan Buddhist monks. He was interested in seeing for himself, and bringing back to his scientific colleagues, manifestations of the concept that the body responds to the power of the mind. In his many publications, Dr. Benson has described his excitement, as well as the sheer power of what he has discovered, on these expeditions.

On one of Dr. Benson's expeditions, it was documented that in forty-degree-Fahrenheit weather the monks could place icy, wet sheets on their naked bodies and then meditate. Within three to five minutes of applying the huge, dripping sheets to their skin, the sheets began to actually produce steam. Within thirty to forty minutes, the sheets were dried completely! The monks were practicing a yoga called "fierce woman" or heat yoga. In this meditative state, the monks were deeply relaxed. Then, through imagery, they envisioned an inner column of heat, from the top of their head through the core of their bodies. They believed this heat was drawn from the universe at large and burned away impurities of the mind and body. Their experience provides an example of how the body follows the mind, why focused thought can produce a tangible physical response, and how strong a "belief system" really is. Also documented and measured was oxygen consumption by the body during the monks' meditation. It was discovered that the monks experienced extraordinarily low rates of oxygen consumption, or metabolism, during this "altered state." [2]

Many new discoveries have followed, and new avenues of research have opened up in this field. In the late 1980s Dr. Benson founded Harvard's Mind/Body Institute, the first in the country. He has continued his research and has written on the subjects of relaxation response, wellness, and healing. Since this break-through research, many mind-body institutes have been established, and there are now numerous mind-body practitioners.

The concept of mind-body medicine has evolved continuously over the last twenty-five years. It has been defined as "holistic medicine"—embracing the human being as a whole and using the entire spectrum of available treatments. It has also been called "alternative medicine," giving it the more political spin of "choice" verses "traditional" therapies. Currently, the more acceptable term is "integrated medicine," evoking collaboration with the joining of different therapies. In addition, over the last five years, a spiritual component has been added, creating the third spoke of the wheel with mind-body-spirit medicine. The mind-body concept has rippled across every aspect of our daily lives. We see it in TV commercials, in special sections in the newspaper, even in how we decorate our homes (feng shui). The world at large has finally accepted that the mind-body connection is an important part of our health and well being. Our society is rediscovering that listening to "the small voice within" is the way to overcome many difficult and unwanted situations in life.

Mind-Body Medicine
(For the Left-Brained Person)

"IMAGES ARE EVENTS TO THE BODY."

-Belleruth Naparstek

THE TERM "mind-body" can bring about a negative response to some people because of its potential association with the extremes of the New Age movement. The new terminology is psychoneuroimmunology (PNI). PNI is the rapidly growing field of science that explores the complex interaction between the neurological system, the immune system, and the endocrine systems, in a word, their "intercommunication." It studies the brain's effect on immune cells and behavior's effect on the immune system. The new discipline of PNI is at the point where the correlation of smoking and cancer was in the 1960s. Research has shown that there is a link between stress and disease, and now scientists are figuring out the mechanisms. The term comes from the concept of interplay between messenger molecules called neurotransmitters (e.g., endorphins, norepinepherine) emitted by the brain and the lyphokines released from the immune system cells. The receptor sites on these specific cells fit these messenger molecules like a key fits into a lock, thereby triggering either the healing activity or the unhealthy response. The psychological piece comes from the important underlying idea in PNI that stress, overall, is much more harmful to the body than we previously realized. We now know that in response to stress, the body releases into the blood stream chemicals that can actually harm the immune system's response to disease.

Stress is a byproduct of work, school, and family—something we all experience in today's fast-paced world. Children are especially susceptible to its harmful influences. Researchers have found that children worry about more than just their friendships, toys, and clothes. They also worry about their parents becoming ill, getting divorced, and being angry, in addition to global issues. Like adults, children now worry about the environment, crime, and wars.

New research shows how chronic stress breaks down the body, making it susceptible to disease. In the short term, the "fight or flight" response was vital to survival, enabling the caveman to walk among saber-toothed tigers without becoming extinct. In the state of "fight or flight," the body activates resources for strength and speed in response to a perceived threat. The brain perceives a threat and a message travels down the spinal cord to the adrenal glands. The adrenal glands secrete adrenaline, the pupils dilate for better vision, the respiratory rate increases to bring in more oxygen, stored sugar is released as glucose into the bloodstream, and the heart rate increases, pumping these fuels to power the body. The cortex of the brain releases cortisol, and the spleen provides extra red blood cells, thereby allowing better use of oxygen. The process of digestion stops, allowing the muscles to receive more energy; the brain dulls the body's sense of pain; thinking is improved.

This all happens in a matter of seconds, making our entire being ready to respond to a warning. If stress becomes chronic, i.e., the "fight or flight" response is activated too frequently, it can negatively affect the heart, brain, and the immune system. Today our stress response is triggered with the morning alarm clock and sustained throughout our day with many stressful circumstances. The response still happens, but the complex mechanisms now cause harm instead of saving a life or limb. It has been shown that brain cells become toxic from sustained cortisol levels, resulting in depression, chronic fatigue, and decreased thinking abilities. The immune system becomes suppressed and cannot resist infection. Blood pressure and heart rate both become chronically elevated, which causes damage to the blood vessels.

With researchers focusing on lifestyle and on social and psychological issues, as well as on physical issues, the holistic approach to medicine is again being brought to the forefront. The good news is that through research it is now accepted, on a concrete scientific level, that the body has an innate ability to self-repair, maintain health, and overcome disease. The key is in becoming aware of this physical ability, understanding the emotional component, and then tapping into the body's inner resources. There are many modalities in the field of PNI now recognized and practiced by physicans, psychiatrists, nurses, and other practitioners. Reiki, therapeutic massage/touch, Interactive Guided Imagery[SM], aromatherapy, herbal medicine, and acupuncture are very popular and are gaining increased respect in the practice of medicine today.

Nurses have always practiced a holistic approach to patient care, and many are now on the forefront of the integrated medicine revolution, as they are the people actually at the patient's bedside, taking care of the patient's needs, and treating the whole person.

PNI has given a scientific basis to holistic medicine, and this has made it "legitimate" to both the public and the medical establishment. In the past, practitioners of traditional medicine had dismissed the holistic approach as "not proven." Now with the vast amount of research done in the PNI field, it can no longer be dismissed.

In mind-body medicine, guided imagery is another of the modalities that is getting more attention of late. Andrew Weil, M.D., associate director of the Integrated Medicine Program at the University of Arizona in Tucson, where he practices natural and preventive medicine, and author of many bestsellers, including *Spontaneous Healing*, endorses guided imagery wholeheartedly. He says, "I find the method so useful that I require that all the Fellows at the Program in Integrated Medicine at the University of Arizona Medical Center learn this technique."[3]

In research studies on directive or guided imagery, Jeff Roman, Ph.D., director of Behavioral Health Medicine at Canyon Ranch in the Berkshires in Massachusetts, conducted a study with sixteen staff

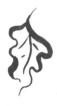

members as part of a general behavioral/educational program for weight loss. One half of the group used an imagery weight loss tape with guided imagery; the other half listened to music. The group that only listened to the imagery weight loss tape (daily) while attending an eight-week weight loss reduction program lost an average of 8.5 pounds. The group that only listened to music while participating in the same weight loss program lost an average of 4.2 pounds.

Alice Domar, Ph.D., director of women's health at Boston's Deaconess Hospital, and co-author with Henry Dreher of *Healing Mind, Healthy Woman*, found that while 20 percent of infertile women got pregnant with standard medical treatment, 57 percent did so when their regimen included support groups, anger management, and guided imagery.[4]

The Relaxation Response
(The Launch Pad of Imagery)

"SO GREAT THE POWER OF THE SOUL UPON THE BODY, THAT WHICHEVER WAY THE SOUL IMAGINES AND DREAMS, THITHER DOTH IT LEAD THE BODY."

–Agrippa

A CRITICAL PIECE of the imagery process is the role of relaxation and the focused mind. A state of relaxed focus enhances the effectiveness of the imagery process by making the child or teen more open and sensitive to the unconscious mind.

First though, imagine our relaxation: imagine a truly relaxed person. Is it possible? The answer is yes. It can be attained with a simple commitment to practice, and, as I have said before, an open heart. This is not to say that becoming fully relaxed is not a challenge in our complex and active lives. A focused, quiet mind is more powerful and ready for the imagery experience. By clearing the mind of clutter you are better able to cope, maintain a sense of peace, and achieve inner balance. At this point, relaxation and a meditative state are not for enlightenment but for healing. That is why I call the relaxation response, or the relaxed state of mind, the launch pad of imagery.

In the early 1970s, after researching the effects of transcendental meditation and its effects on hypertension Dr. Benson coined the phrase "the relaxation response." He found that "the body has an inborn capacity to enter a special state characterized by lowered heart rate, decreased rate of breathing, lowered blood pressure, slower brain waves, and an overall reduction of the speed of metabolism." These alpha brain waves are found when the right side of the brain is activated, counterbalancing the fight or flight response (stimulating the parasympathetic nervous system). The relaxation response is the natural, healing phenomenon that can change your physiology and improve health by using your mind. Relaxation causes an altered state, one that is focused, energized, alert, and deeply sensitive. The creative right brain is where the in-depth work of imagery occurs, making it possible for the small voice within to be heard. This psycho-physiological condition allows us to communicate with the "inner self," drawing on the body's and the mind's internal wisdom and making us more capable of insight and self-healing. Younger children are not usually aware of these complex mechanisms. Some older children or teenagers will begin to understand these more complex concepts. As a parent, you can explain and discuss ideas and intuitions as you both go further into the imagery process, discovering new and exciting conceptions.[5]

The relaxation response can be elicited in several ways, by using a number of mind-focusing techniques such as deep breathing, a repetitive sound or word, meditation, and head-to-toe muscle relaxation exercises. It is up to the parent-child team to decide which technique or combination of techniques work for them. To increase the effectiveness of the relaxation response, it is recommended to practice for ten to twenty minutes, once or twice a day.

The challenge for both parent and child in using relaxation techniques is to fit them into today's busy lifestyle. This is one of the most important issues: making time for oneself and for wellness. As with any physical or mental activity, consistent practice reinforces its effectiveness.

At Harvard's Mind/Body Institute, researchers have created a concept they call "minis" or "bite-size versions of the relaxation response." Minis are a way to evoke the relaxation response quickly during a stressful event or for the mere benefits that it produces in the body (e.g., dropping your blood pressure down a few points). Taking a deep breath, using a trigger (word or anchor), and letting go of the tension can do it. Later, we will look at another tecnique—recall.

What Is a Placebo?

"... [S]OME PATIENTS, THOUGH CONSCIOUS THAT
THEIR CONDITION IS PERILOUS, RECOVER THEIR
HEALTH SIMPLY THROUGH THEIR CONTENTMENT
WITH THE GOODNESS OF THE PHYSICIAN."

-Hippocrates

PLACEBO comes from the Latin phrase, "I shall please." The definition of a placebo is a medication prescribed more for the mental relief of the patient than for its actual effect on a disorder. It can be an inert or innocuous substance such as sugar tablets, used especially in controlled experiments testing the efficacy of another substance, or it can be something intended to soothe the patient.

What better way to think of healing imagery than to soothe?

The potential of the human brain is immense, and many scientists worldwide have dedicated their lives to the study of its capabilities. I want to touch on one of the most fascinating of these studies: the placebo effect. The placebo effect is the improvement in the condition of a sick person in response to "treatment" with no specific correlation to the specific treatment.

This particular effect has intrigued scientists, physicians, and philosophers for thousands of years. There has been a resurgence in the study of the placebo effect over the last two to three decades. This interest has led many practitioners as well as laymen to embrace its use. Now apparent is the power the mind has over the body—the ways our personal beliefs and mental activity affect the body. We make it well with positive thoughts and unwell with worried and negative thoughts. Simply, the placebo effect happens when we believe that we are receiving the "right" treatment and we become well. Conversely, if you believe that you are not receiving the best treatment, then you may become more ill. In America, some HMOs are now covering spiritual counseling because they are realizing that health care is about more than just the treatment of physical symptoms. They are now focusing on the whole well-being of their members.

These are simple examples to show how your mind affects your body, but beyond these discoveries comes an even more fascinating concept of "faith." The simple trust and belief you hold in your doctor or caregiver can produce a positive outcome in your health. This is the basis of Eastern medicine. A physician's kindness, reassurances, karma, and concern affect each and every one of his or her patients. Their relationship is built on trust alone, and that feeling of trust by itself can virtually produce healing. Placebos are given to patients from the Himalayan Mountains, in the islands of Fiji, and on 5th Avenue in New York City. The trusting and respected relationship between the practitioner and the patient is paramount to a positive outcome.

Health care providers other than physicians affect their patients. Without exception, nurse, lab technicians, and X-ray technicians have the same aftereffect on each person they tend to. Scientists have made evident that the role of belief, trust, and faith in one's physician plays an important part in recovery and response to treatment. I have found that the attitude of the parent to the child plays an equally important role. The following two scenarios are both the positive and the negative sides of parental influence that I have witnessed as a practitioner of guided imagery.

My seven-year-old daughter was complaining of symptoms of conjunctivitis at bedtime. She had yellow drainage oozing from both eyes and was complaining of itch and discomfort. I knew what this meant—another trip to the doctor's in the morning. Naturally, we used imagery to help her block some of her symptoms and get to sleep. After initiating relaxation, she went to her special place and brought forward the image of her inner advisor, Freddie the raccoon. Freddie had introduced her to many different guides, but this night he introduced her to Dr. Porky, a porcupine—and the forest's doctor! After the introductions were done, my daughter went on to ask Dr. Porky for his help. He immediately went to work and got a pod and filled it with mixed leaves, grass, river water, and other things from the woods to make a salve. He then gently put the salve on her eyes, and she fell asleep immediately. The next morning she was completely symptom free. I was truly astounded, checking her all day, not a symptom to be found! I witnessed the disappearance of objective, measurable symptoms due to the power of her faith in the imagery process and the placebo effect.

I also have a contrary example to share. I was introducing imagery to a twelve-year-old child to help her decrease the pain of her migraine headaches. She was very interested and engaged in the explanation of imagery and how it worked. A standard statement in my introduction is, "this will work," which begins to establish the placebo effect as well as the belief in self-healing. Before we started, I asked the mother (and the child) if she wanted to stay, and they both agreed to have the mother stay during the initial session. The mother stated that she had chronic back pain and wanted to see if imagery could also help her. The imagery session went very well for the little girl, making her relaxed and pain free! As we wrapped up the session, grounding the experience through discussion, the mother suddenly announced that the session did "nothing" for her back pain. I was shocked. Part of my practice is establishing a trust with each child, conveying the positives of the imagery process, and trying to instill a belief in me as a practitioner as well as in the imagery process. I sat there waiting to see what would happen next. As we continued to wrap up the session, the little girl started to complain about headache pain. Her enthusiasm had diminished, and I could see I was losing her. Her mother's negative words and attitude affected her mind and, therefore, her body.

On subsequent visits when the child requested that the mother wait in the waiting room, she was able to get great benefit from the imagery session. When her mother stayed with us, the session was not as successful.

Three: *The Heart of the Matter*

"WHAT GIFT HAS PROVIDENCE BESTOWED ON MAN
THAT IS SO DEAR TO HIM AS HIS CHILDREN."

–Cicero

THE ROLE of the parent as guide is an important one.
I have found that understanding this role is one of the
most crucial steps in starting imagery with a sick child.
Your own feelings and beliefs as parent or caretaker have
an impact on the imagery process as a whole. Children
are very perceptive to other people's negative moods and
feelings, or to signs of tension or insincerity. They will
instinctively sense these attitudes and may not respond
well to guided imagery. This goes back to the placebo
effect and to how belief and trust affect healing. To overcome this problem, you may first want to take the time
to do a personal, simple imagery session for yourself, to
get a sense of what imagery is about and what feelings it
brings out for you. This preparation is key to the process
and will help you relate to the imagery process on an
intimate level, making it much more comfortable to be in
the role of the parent-turned-imagery-guide. Any personal experience expands one's understanding and can be
a real "attitude fixer" as well as "fear reducer." It also helps
you to trust the process yourself.

Another important aspect of using imagery with
your child or teen is parental style. Your particular style
and how it affects your child should be examined at the

beginning and then periodically throughout this process. With illness or injury, both you and your child experience a multitude of emotions: fear, anger, exhaustion, relief, happiness, self-doubt, and denial, to name a few. They are each much different from each other.

Remember your child is different from you. For parents of the chronically ill, accepting the understanding that your child is different can be difficult, but embracing this concept is certainly worth it, bringing insight to "the long haul" of chronic illness. I prefer the word "special" child in place of "different." As parent and child, you have experienced the same situations—emergencies, hospitalizations, new medications, difficult procedures, and everyday symptoms. Diagnoses vary, but similar issues are raised for you both, and you each experience them differently. The point here is simply just to realize this difference and refocus on it occasionally, embracing the differences between your style and your child's style of interpreting and coping. Your role as the guide does not include interpreter. Once again, accept the child as an individual, and honor that individualism as a parent.

Be aware that not all people imagine in the same way. Many people feel a presence, or sense a shape or light. These wonderful people we call "kinesthetics" or image-less imagers. Kinetics is the science of motion. These children may feel a presence or have a "feeling" instead of a mind-picture during imagery. Not to worry, it just makes things more interesting! Go about the imagery sessions as you normally would with special attention to these feelings and what they represent. They can speak as strongly as anything can visually.

As part of an imagery program for nurses (called Beyond Ordinary Nursing), the nursing process is used to delineate the three major steps in an imagery session. The following review of those steps can be helpful to parents as well as to the medical practitioner.

The first step is "assessment." This is when much of the initial or general information about the child is gathered, most of which the parent already knows. As a parent, look at assessment as an opportunity to find out something you may have not known about the situation, some small missing piece that will bring further insight to you as a parent as well as a guide. During assessment, you should go over the steps in the session: the type of relaxation, the imagery script that is to be read, or the interactive technique that is to be used, and finally the coming back process. It is also important to establish the means by which you two will communicate. I ask children to lift a finger or nod their head when they are ready for the next step. Additionally, the child or teen should have a way to tell you if he or she has a problem or concern of some kind during the imagery. This is the point where you can clarify any misgivings or misunderstandings about the process and identify any other preferences the child may have. Much information can be collected during this initial step through body language and your understanding of the child's previous experiences. You as the guide will be gathering information from all of the child's senses. You know your child, so these subtle clues should be easy to identify, but keeping notes is a good habit.

The next step is "intervention," which includes the induction of the relaxation response and imagery. Intervention is the place where the child does his or her inner exploration work. Through sensory recruitment, you as a parent/guide facilitate a type of communication between the child and the images. This communication is essential with both guided imagery that is read from this book, or in Interactive Guided Imagery™, in which the imagery becomes active for the child or teen. This step is also where you honor your child's "sacred space" while you give all the time your child needs.

The last step is "evaluation" and "wrap-up." This is a time of review, reflection, and grounding, giving time for the child to draw or write about the imagery. The "wrap-up" follows each Interactive Imagery™ session with several questions you may want to ask your child. This is a time for you to listen and not interpret. If your child does not want to write or draw, you may want to jot down pertinent information in the blank note area provided. These notes will help you to remember details of the experience, such as body language and the names of certain images. You might gently probe for information about your child's experience and feelings at the conclusion of the imagery session, always keeping in mind that it is the child's process, not yours. Give your child time to talk, respectfully staying silent. Let the child interpret or voice the experience . . . in the child's own way!

In wrap up, the parent can discuss any concerns, feelings, or conflicts the child may have experienced. It is also a good time to check in with the child on the method used. Ask questions like these: "Did you like the imagery?" "Would a different color or relaxation technique be preferred?" "Was it helpful?" "Do you want to try a different imagery?" Always avoid interpreting the experience for the child. You are guiding the child to shine some light on a particular problem and are assisting the child to find the answers for himself or herself. You and your child can then establish a plan of practice. Usually a daily imagery session for fifteen to thirty minutes is helpful for most symptoms, with recall as needed. The beauty of recall is it can be used throughout the day, anytime, anywhere.

Be aware that this imagery does work in stressful situations, provided you stay calm and in control of the situation. In an emergency, a powerful, directed imagery could prevent an escalation of the stress for both you and your child in an emergency. I have used this technique for years while working in the emergency room, for it is especially helpful when a child requires suturing or a bone set. Though children are crying and frightened, I have been able to help them relax somewhat (which decreased their fear and pain) and then go on to do directed imagery. This technique enables them to endure the procedure. They have the power, through imagery, to be better in control of their bodies and of the situation.

Parent as a Guide

"WHEN YOU TALK YOU REPEAT WHAT YOU ALREADY
KNOW; WHEN YOU LISTEN, YOU OFTEN LEARN
SOMETHING."

-Anonymous

AS A GUIDE you will act as the bridge for your child to
cross over into the imagination and the inner self. You will
guide your child or teen to explore individual symptoms
and situations, thus encouraging insight to your child's
feelings about them. Your bridge will support your child
while he or she begins to recognize any special needs and
to develop a respect for the child's innermost feelings. As
the guide, you will help to stimulate your child's abilities
in self-exploration and self-expression while developing a
deep sense of trust—not only in you as a parent, but more
important, a sense of self-trust. This trust and insight
help your child to solve problems, which is essential to
self-healing. With this support and trust, your child will
begin to relax and explore the inner self, hearing the small
voice within. This is the point where the imagery starts to
work, becoming actual events for the body.

I have also found that imagery helps you as a parent
(of an ill child) to get some needed distance from a difficult situation and bring a new and fresh perspective to
it. There is an old Chinese proverb that says, "You can
pick up the world, but can you put it down?"

You will find that acting as the bridge in the
imagery process is an important and rewarding role for

you as the parent. As you learn the techniques of imagery, both guided and Interactive Guided Imagery^{SM}, you will also learn to be a better listener. You will learn when to be silent. You will begin to believe in things that may not be concrete and explainable. You may have flashes of feeling like a child again.

Journal Writing

"WHEN IDEAS FAIL, WORDS COME IN VERY HANDY."
–Johann Wolfgang von Goethe

KEEPING A JOURNAL can help express feelings and thoughts about an experience as well as ground that experience. In imagery, both the parent and child can keep a personal journal. It does not have to be complicated or difficult. It is just another tool to help the child better understand and express personal experiences with imagery, stress, coping, illness, and/or injury. With imagery, all the senses are stimulated, producing an extraordinary picture overall. This picture brings the child or teen to a place of openness, ready to start understanding the inner self and all its wisdom. Writing is another way to connect the outer self to the inner self.

Select a journal that will be comfortable and easy to use. Read what you have written after writing it. This re-reading helps to ground it. It is best if you do not limit your styles. Try using poetry, drawings, and other forms of expression. It does not matter if it is "good" writing or not—that is not the point. Certainly don't worry about grammar or spelling. Also remember that neither you nor your child has to share a journal. Children usually do want to share, but teenagers are most likely to want privacy concerning their writings and drawings. This desire for privacy should be completely honored by the parent or caregiver.

Research has shown that journal writing can have a profound effect on our mental and physical well-being. The Journal of the American Medical Association published a study by the North Dakota State University's psychiatric department. Professor Joshua M. Smyth found that journal writing could improve physical symptoms. Researchers recruited 112 women and men with the chronic diseases of arthritis and asthma and studied them over a period of four months. Half of the patients were to write in their journal on neutral subjects and the other half on very stressful events that had occurred in their lives. Each group did twenty minutes of writing on three consecutive days. Smyth and his associates found that the asthma patients who wrote about the negative, painful events in their lives improved their lung function by 19 percent, and the patients that wrote about benign events had no improvement at all. The collating arthritis patients experienced a decrease in disease severity by 28 percent, compared with no change for the patients who wrote on neutral subjects. Though the research is not complete, Professor Smyth theorizes that writing about traumatic events may have helped the participants to finally deal with their misfortune and suffering and to come to a place of acceptance. This acceptance, in turn, decreased the stress symptoms that were affecting their overall health and well-being.[6]

Body language is subtle but very informative. As the guide, you have time to watch your child during the imagery session. Once you are tuned into body language, it is an amazing and revealing form of communication. You will notice smiling, grimacing, body tightening, laughing, and changing posture while the child is imaging. If the child becomes distressed, simply discontinue the session, quickly and quietly, and then debrief. This book gives you blank note areas for making notes on these details. You will find that notes will assist you in your future sessions.

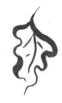

What About Breathing?

"BREATH IS THE ESSENCE OF BEING."

-Dr. Andrew Weil

THROUGHOUT THE CENTURIES and in a multitude of cultures, the act of focused breathing is intricately linked with relaxation and meditation. Breathing has been an important part of becoming relaxed, both physically and mentally. This link, in turn, makes breathing important to the imagery experience. It has been found that restricted breathing can reduce the efficiency of our metabolism, leading to a decrease in how our healing system operates. For our purposes, the basics of relaxed, focused breathing will be discussed. If you would like more in-depth information on meditative breathing techniques, books on the art of breathing fill bookstores today.

Children can do deep breathing in a focused way with some simple instruction. Both you and your child should begin by getting into a position of comfort, either lying down or sitting erect in a chair. Softly shut your eyes and "feel" or imagine a smile on your face even though you are not smiling. I usually point out the nature of a "regular" breath, which is how we all breathe while going through our day, using the mid-chest. Then I point out the "scared" breath, which is upper-chest breathing—shallow, restricted, and rapid. The "scared" breath has a purpose, which is part of the flight or fight survival mechanism. Breathing affects our central nervous system in both positive and negative ways. Mid-chest and upper-chest breathing is not useful in deepening relaxation. I then go on to demonstrate what is called "belly breathing": placing the hands over the abdomen and breathing slowly in through the nose, expanding the belly outward on inhalation and deflating it on exhalation. This is diaphragmatic breathing. It works well if you have the child lie down and place a little stuffed animal on the middle of the stomach. It gives a concrete measure on how to make the stomach rise and fall while breathing. Try to keep the breathing continuous without a beginning or an end. Bring all the attention to the breath and only the breath. Let thoughts freely enter the mind and leave the mind, paying no attention to them, returning to the breath. This type of breathing does take practice, so do not get discouraged. Maintain the practice of relaxed breathing, and it will become an intricate part of your child's or teen's daily well-being. Do a relaxation exercise like this prior to doing an imagery activity.

Imagery Exercise for the Parent

"SOON THE CHILD'S CLEAR EYE IS CLOUDED OVER BY IDEAS AND OPINIONS, PREOCCUPATIONS AND ABSTRACTIONS. SIMPLE FREE BEING BECOMES ENCRUSTED WITH THE BURDENSOME ARMOR OF THE EGO. NOT UNTIL YEARS LATER DOES AN INSTINCT COME THAT A VITAL SENSE OF MYSTERY HAS BEEN WITHDRAWN. . . . AFTER THAT DAY . . . WE BECOME SEEKERS."

–Peter Matthiessen

I HAVE FOUND that the best way to be a good guide for a child is to be informed and comfortable with the imagery process. Before doing imagery with your child, try an imagery exercise for yourself. Your initial, personal imagery session introduces you to the experience of relaxation and to the sensations and insights of imagery itself. The session does not have to be complicated or lengthy. Just take your time and enjoy and learn from the experience. It is an important exercise because it makes you familiar with the steps in imagery, helping you to become a more insightful and receptive guide for your child's sessions.

First, if you do not have your own relaxation techniques in place, you may want to reread the section in chapter 2 called "The Relaxation Response" (p. 26). Set the stage by creating a quiet, comfortable environment, with the telephone shut off and no extraneous noises (such as a TV in the background) to distract you. You can do the exercise in silence, but it is fine to have some soothing, soft music playing. Many people find an aromatic candle enhances the relaxation experience. The point is just to slow down.

To start, take time to clear the mind of the chatter of the day, becoming comfortable (loose comfortable clothes are a must). Now create the relaxation response with slow, focused, deep breathing. For our purposes, the focus is to remain with the breath, going back to it each time a thought enters into your mind. Let go of thought and simply return the mind to your breathing. There is no need to count the breaths or be caught up trying to do it right. What is right is what works for you.

Once you have completed a few minutes of focused breathing—perhaps ten deep, focused breaths—begin to relax the body with a simple head-to-toe relaxation. It can be enjoyable to have a spouse or trusted friend read the following relaxation exercise for you; this practice will show you how the process will work when you do it with your child. Other options are to do it by yourself after reading this written relaxation, or to record yourself reading it. Any way is perfectly acceptable. In the following is a head-to-toe relaxation exercise.

RELAXATION TECHNIQUES

(Read, slowly paced)

CLOSE your eyes and begin to relax ... letting go of the tension in your body ... letting go of stressful thoughts.... You have nowhere to go and nothing to do.... As you breathe out, let any tension you may have leave your body with the breath ... breathing out tension and stress, breathing in peace and relaxation ... going inward ... centering yourself ... inwardly smile ... start with the top of your head, and imagine a warm luminous light entering through the crown of your head.... Let this warm, relaxing light melt over your entire scalp ... releasing and softening it.... Continue to focus on this warm light as it melts over your face ... softening and removing tension from your entire face ... softening the eyes ... relaxing the jaw ... letting your mouth and jaw become slack.... Let the luminous light travel to your throat and hold it there ... filling that area.... Place your hand to your throat.... This is where emotions are held.... Let it become soft, quiet.... Let the swirling warm light travel down the back of the head into the neck...releasing each vertebra of the neck ... running down the neck to the shoulders ...releasing and softening...opening each shoulder ... let this warm luminous light melt and swirl down both your arms ... to the elbows and then to the wrists ... softening.... It fills each finger.... Your hands are heavy, warm, and thick. Go back to the top of your spine.... Let the warm swirl travel...filling the wing bones and back with warmth and relaxation ... travelling down the entire spine ... release and soften each vertebra.... Go back to the front of your body and take a deep cleansing breath...breathing the luminous light into your chest.... Let its warm, healing light wrap around your heart and hold it there [place your hand over your heart area].... Another deep breath and pull the light into your belly ... softening and relaxing it.... Let it flow down into each hip ... opening each hip joint ... softening.... The entire upper half of your body is relaxed and comfortable.... Allow the warm feeling to cover the entire pelvis and buttock area ... flowing down each leg ... softening and releasing tension.... Let each knee joint open.... Let the ankles and feet follow.... Image the light blazing out of the soles of your feet.... Check to see if there is any leftover tension in the body, and go back to it, and breathe into that area ... letting go of the tension ... relaxing the area. Your body is light and edgeless.

Now go to your "special place," that place you can go to in your mind, anytime, anyplace. It is a place of beauty, safety, and peace. It can be someplace totally imagined or a place you are familiar with. I have found that letting the image just come, rather than consciously creating it, works well. But this is your process, so let your unconscious mind help you get here. The image or feeling of a special place can come to you slowly or immediately. Don't worry if it takes a while. Stay relaxed, and an image or an essence of a special place will come. And remember to trust the process. The image or feeling of a special place will come! (Please refer to "the special place" written script on p. 110)

When you try to imagine a special place, many images may flash through your mind at once. You may feel as if you have to control this flood of images, but don't. Let the images flash through, and, eventually, one will stay in your mind's eye.

COMING BACK FROM AN IMAGERY EXERCISE

KEEP YOURSELF relaxed and quiet, returning slowly to the room you are in. Gradually awaken, feeling your body heavy and comfortable, but slowly beginning to lighten. You are back in the room where you started, and you are now fully alert. Do not sit up quickly if you have been lying down. Do it in stages, slowly rising. Once you are fully alert, drink a glass of water to ground your body, physically.

Grounding: If you wish, take some time to write your feelings, observations, and insights in response to this imagery exercise. Some people prefer to draw a picture of their image or the experience, which is certainly acceptable. As previously discussed, this "journaling" helps you to gather your thoughts and remember them, so use the area below for any personal notes. You may also find that insights and thoughts come to you hours or days after the exercise. Jot down anything you feel is pertinent or helpful.

Note Area

Note Area

Note Area

Four: Guided Imagery

"IMAGINATION IS MORE IMPORTANT THAN
KNOWLEDGE. KNOWLEDGE IS LIMITED. IMAGINATION
ENCIRCLES THE WORLD."
                                        -Albert Einstein

To ENHANCE their performances, athletes for many
years have used powerful mind exercises known as
visualizations. Through visualization, the runner, foot-
ball player, or skater is able to preview the performance, experience it, meditating on it. It is also a way
for the athletes to review and evaluate their performance, so they can improve upon it. But the athletes
do not just visualize their performance. They feel it in
every way, as if they were there. They are able to reach
that altered state of alert focus. They call this altered
state "The Zone." What they are really doing
is imagery!

Guided imagery is a form of directive meditation,
similar to visualization, except that it takes in all the
senses, not just vision. You feel, smell, and hear the
experience, while listening to scripted, directive
imagery provided for you by a practitioner or on audiotape. Many guided imagery tapes are available for
specific conditions from smoking cessation to labor
pain control.

In *Guided Imagery for Healing Children and Teens*,
there are many scripted, guided imageries for you to use,

some for specific symptoms such as fever reduction and pain relief. These written, directive imageries have been used with very small children as well as with the adolescents, with great results. The younger children enjoy the storybook type of tale, while naturally the written imagery for teenagers is a bit more sophisticated and "cool." I tell them that it's like going to the movies but in your head. Guided imagery adds sensory recruitment to the story, which draws the child in, helping the child actually to experience the story with the senses. Remember the example of the lemon and how it can increase salivation? The images of wellness and healing, love, and joy can be made just as real, felt just as strongly by the body and the mind. Reading imagery is an excellent way to become familiar with the imagery process, and it is a great "ice breaker" and starting point with a child or teen.

Guided imagery also works beautifully if a child or teenager is extremely ill or experiencing severe pain. Being able to evoke a sense of peacefulness and love works wonders with anyone, ill or otherwise. Recognize this truth and honor it. These children would simply like to listen to a story that provides some relaxation, some stress relief, and some diminished symptoms. The teens I have worked with like guided imagery when they are feeling overwhelmed and want to step out of their role as teenager and embrace the feeling of being a child again.

How to Start (For the Child)

"THERE ARE NO DAYS IN LIFE SO MEMORABLE AS
THOSE WHICH VIBRATED TO SOME STROKE OF THE
IMAGINATION."

-Ralph Waldo Emerson

THE BEGINNING is similar to the parent's personal prep session. To start, you (the parent or caregiver as guide) should be relaxed before starting a guided imagery session with a child, taking the time for deep breathing to become calm. Again, keep in mind that a child or teen is very receptive to the moods and emotions of the parents.

Both you and your child should be comfortably dressed and in relaxed positions. Before reading a healing imagery narrative for the first time to your child, take some time to explain the imagery process. Keep it simple and brief, but answer any questions your child may have. Using the blank note areas in the book, write down anything you notice about your child's ideas, preferences, or likes and dislikes concerning the course of the imagery. Explain that you will be asking the child to hear, smell, taste, and touch things during the imagery, so they know it is okay and part of the practice.

It is difficult to convey the imagery experience in words the first time, so doing a brief session is usually the way to start, incorporating a "show of power." Remember that this step is simply showing the child or teenager that he or she can image. Keep it simple; it should not to get too complicated.

Once you and your child have set up a loosely structured landscape for the session, you can begin.

Tell your child to close the eyes softly and start to breathe, deeply and slowly (see the following exercise). They do not have to count or do the breathing "correctly." A quiet, concentrated focus on breathing will do the trick. Thoughts and ideas will continue to occur, but tell the child to let these thoughts float away when they appear and to concentrate back to the breath, which is the classic approach to meditation. I have found even the youngest of children can do slow, deep breathing very well with guidance.

For some children, a lavender-scented, flaxseed eye pack is soothing for the eyes, and helps them to keep their eyes shut. If children do not want to shut their eyes, they can choose a focal point. A focal point can be anything in the room that they can continuously look at to focus their attention. It can be anything already in the room or something particularly special. A colorful drawing, a toy, or flower can act as a focal point. Let the children be involved in the decisions to create the imagery to look and "feel" the way they wish. You and your child can discuss and adjust any particular needs or want, so get creative!

The environment for relaxation and imagery is one of calm, peace, intimacy, and trust. It helps to have no extraneous sounds (e.g., TV), and low lighting always enhances the onset of relaxation. Keep your voice monotone and slow paced. There is no rush. In both guided and Interactive Imagery^{SM}, "mirror" the child's words rather than "interpreting" them during an imagery session. Another handy technique is just saying, "go on" or "tell me more," always keeping the communication open and flowing. This openness helps you as the guide to stay focused and remain detached (it's not your process). I find it keeps you in a state of patient listening rather than speaking, a state that is essential for the child's own course of imagery.

The Magic of Touch

"YOU, YOURSELF, AS MUCH AS ANYBODY IN THE ENTIRE UNIVERSE, DESERVE YOUR LOVE AND AFFECTION."
—*Buddha*

THE NEXT STEP is self-massage of the face (see the following exercise), but first a few words on the power of touch. Touch has been proven to be an important aspect of the healing process. Simple touch for a newborn baby promotes well-being in that child. It can help to decrease a racing heart rate or increase blood flow to the brain. Children held and touched since birth have fewer emotional and psychological problems and fewer learning disabilities later in life. Therapeutic massage therapists report that while they are performing a healing massage, many clients respond by experiencing vivid and powerful images. Memories of forgotten events are somehow stimulated by the touch of a trained specialist. Touch is one of the triggers that bring these images to the surface, or conscious mind. Touch heals. Therapeutic massage and energy healing techniques are on the rise as alternatives to more traditional therapies.

When performing imagery, the child can touch a certain area of the body to amplify the power of the imagery. Placing a hand over a body part, like the heart or lung area, and then focusing in on that part and its functions strengthens the imagery. You can project particular feelings into a part of the body as well. Often I have the children imagine the feeling of warmth and release in their throat, placing their hand to their throat, while doing the relaxation exercise. The throat holds emotion, as in the "lump in the throat," so I have them concentrate and dissolve this lump and, in turn, dissolve the emotion and discomfort. A diabetic child can place a hand over the pancreas (abdomen) and imagine insulin being made and used by the body. The point is that you can image your cells, the body's blood flow, and all the millions of mechanisms that go on inside your body. You can just as effectively image the healing mechanisms within your body. For example, you can picture your white cells gobbling up a virus, your blood vessels opening and dilating to furnish blood flow to nourish a body part, the matrix of your bone closing a fracture, or nerve endings becoming dull to the sensation of pain. Your body and mind have an immense and untapped power to heal.

Don't be afraid of tears if they come. Both guided imagery and Interactive Imagery[SM] cause a release of emotions, so tears are very common. These tears can come simply from a release of tension, both physical and emotional. Tears are how the body handles these incredible feelings of release. With the obvious emotional component to the imagery, you may have tears of joy or of sadness. The "special place" or an "inner advisor" can bring out intense feelings and emotions. Many times, if an advisor is a long-dead grandmother or if the special place is a family home long gone, it can elicit tears of loss and nostalgia. But more often than not, many children find sensory imagery to be a release of tension and a very empowering experience, which leads to tears of gratitude and happiness. If the child is crying, hang in there a moment, and trust the process. Try not to rescue the child immediately. The crying may be for a reason. Check it out with your child or teen, and see how they explain and interpret their tears.

As you both become comfortable, introduce your child to facial self-massage, an excellent way to relax muscles and let go of tension. You can help by demonstrating it for the child and receiving the benefits of the massage for yourself!

To begin: "Gently massage your forehead . . . getting rid of the worry lines in your brow . . . (slowly) smoothing them out with a sweeping massage ... your worries melting away ... let your fingertips softly massage around your eyes ... going slowly ... pressing around the entire eye ... releasing and softening. ... Gently smooth out the eyebrows ... getting rid of the pressure and strain ... taking your time ... relaxed ... easy ... going on to the cheek and jaw area with circling, soft pressure ... release your face ... enjoy the warm, easy, soft movement of your own hands. ... Go to the jaw bone, where the hinge of your jaw is ... rub in slow circular motions ... (slowly) ... getting rid of all the tension. ... Now move on to your ears ... softly touching and massaging ... to your throat area ... gently massaging ... very lightly. ... Go to your neck area ... rubbing and releasing. ... Go back to any place that stills holds tension or stress and massage and release that tension."

Do this for a few minutes. It is very relaxing and enjoyable for most people. Self-massage is a lovely addition to the relaxation exercise and can easily be incorporated into your personal formula. But keep in mind that anything that does not feel right does not have to be practiced. In other words, there are really no "shoulds" in imagery.

You may want to audio tape any of the exercises in this book. This will give you a way to easily do the imagery with your personal touch, using special colors, names, and feelings.

Relaxation for Children

"AFTER THE VERB 'TO LOVE,' 'TO HELP' IS THE MOST BEAUTIFUL VERB IN THE WORLD."

–Bertha von Suttner

CHILDREN LOVE the head-to-toe relaxation (see p. 47). If you have established a certain color or temperature, use it here. The senses of temperature and color seem to be of particular importance during the relaxation phase. Some children enjoy a warm, luminous light color while others prefer a cool, deep color like blue or purple. Make sure to check it out with your child. The head-to-toe is literally the way this relaxation works, but as you both grow into the process, you can always start to develop your own methods. For instance, you can start at the feet or at the core (heart) of the body and work the relaxation outward from there. It is all about preference, comfort, and enjoyment. Go slowly and pace your reading. Work with your child; make it the child's process. This ownership will start gently to stir the feelings of empowerment and self-healing.

SCRIPT ONE

CLOSE YOUR EYES and begin to relax ... letting go of the tension in your body ... letting go of anything that is bothering you ... you have nowhere to go and nothing to do.... As you breathe in, breathe in quietly, and as you breathe out, let any worry, sadness, or pain, leave your body with the breath ... breathing out tension and stress, breathing in peace and relaxation ... (slowly) ... your inner smile is starting.... Begin with the top of your head, and imagine a warm glowing light entering through the very top of your head ... let this warm, relaxing light melt over your entire scalp, releasing and softening it ... warming your entire head.... Focus on this soft, warm light as it melts over your face ... softening and removing tightness from your entire face ... softening the eyes ... relaxing the jaw ... letting your mouth open slightly.... Let the beautiful light travel to your throat, and hold it there ... filling that area [Have the child place a hand on the throat area].... This is where sadness or stress can live.... Let it become soft, quiet ... continuing to breathe and relax.... Let the swirling, warm, light travel down the back of the head into the neck ... releasing each bone of the neck ... running down the neck to the shoulders ... releasing and softening ... opening each shoulder ... filling the wing bones and back with warmth and relaxation ... the light swirls down both your arms ... lightening them ... melts into each elbow and down to each hand ... your fingers release and soften ... your hands feel warm ... thick and heavy. ... Now go back to the top of your spine ... let the melting light travel down the entire back bone ... releasing and softening. ... Go back to the front of your body and take a deep cleansing breath ... (slowly) ... breathing the luminous light into your chest. ... Let its warm, healing light wrap around your heart and hold it there [Have the child place a hand over the heart area]. ... Another deep breath and pull the light into your belly ... softening and relaxing it. ... Let it flow down into each hip ... opening each hip joint ... softening. ... The entire upper half of your body is relaxed and comfortable. ... Allow the warm feeling to cover the entire hip area ... then into your bottom ... relaxing ... flowing down each leg, softening and releasing tension ... let each knee open ... let the ankles and feet follow ... image the light blazing out of the bottom of your feet. ... You have a glorious beam of healing light that runs through your entire body ...

it starts at the top of your head and goes to the bottoms of your feet.... Check to see if there is any leftover tension in the body and go back to it and breathe into that area... letting go of the tension ... relaxing the area ... you cannot feel anything beneath you ... you are edgeless and feel as if you are floating ... your body heavy with relaxation.

SCRIPT TWO

YOU are lying down on your back.... Start to take slow, deep breaths into your belly. Make your belly bigger as you breathe in, and let it flatten down as you breathe out. [Perhaps the child wants to place a small stuffed animal on his or her belly.] Don't worry about your breathing. Just let it happen. You can feel your whole body begin to relax with each breath ... breathing out stress and worry ... breathing in relaxation and calm. Centering yourself... inwardly smile. Deep breathing, relaxing... now imagine a warm ball of light in your belly. Every time you take a breath in, the warm ball of light climbs up the front of your body, becoming bigger, expanding. It is now in your chest, making it feel warm and light ... with another inhala-

tion, it travels up into your throat and neck ...
each time you breathe in, the warm ball of light
grows bigger ... it is filling you. ... Your face is
now filled with this warm light and your jaw
loosens ... let your mouth open slightly. ... The
ball of light reaches the top of your head ...
relaxing your scalp ... it travels with each inward
breath down the back of your head to your spine
... warming and relaxing your entire back ...
softening each bone in your back. The ball of
light rolls slowly down both arms ... then to
your hands ... making them heavy and warm. ...
This warm flow slowly moves into each of your
legs ... traveling to your knees ... ankles ... softly
on to your feet ... warming you ... each toe and
bone in your foot is relaxed ... softened. This
warm ball of relaxation is in your whole body. It
is everywhere. Keep breathing and let all your
tension and worry be gone ... quiet ... melted
away. Go back to any area that has any tightness
and bring the warm ball of healing light back to
it. Take your time. You are warm, relaxed, happy,
and safe. Your body is heavy and comfortable ...
filled with relaxation.

Once the child is relaxed, quieted, and in a state of
focused alertness, you can read any of the self-healing

imageries. There are relaxation cues in each story to keep the child in a quiet and focused state while you read. It is okay if the child does not want to pick out the imagery that will be read, so go ahead and pick out an imagery that you feel would benefit the situation.

Keep your voice soft, lilting, at a steady volume, and slow paced for both the relaxation and the introduction of the guided imagery. Your voice can become more animated when the imagery requires it (i.e., when the Blue Whales battle the Frownies). Imagery may look passive in nature, but it is actually an active experience. You will notice that many of the endings have a triumph of good overcoming bad, so it is perfectly appropriate to read it as you would a fairy tale. Mixing the styles together is a plus. The pace is slow and flowing. With some of the written imagery, if you return to a softer voice toward the end, this softness will subtly signal that you are coming to the end, and it's time to return to a more relaxed state. When the reading is complete, let the child remain quiet and focused. Let the inner processes work.

Your child may fall asleep. What do you do? This happens especially when first starting the imagery process. The first or second time, let it go; be thankful your child is able to become relaxed and tension free. But self-healing needs an awake mind. The child in the altered state of relaxation is open, alert, and focused. This is the optimum state for healing imagery to occur and become beneficial. The child could sit up during the first imagery session and keep eyes open. With practice, any problem with sleepiness should correct itself. I have never had it continue to be a prolonged problem with any of my patients.

Have the child return slowly to the room, gradually awakening, coming back. The child should not open his or her eyes too quickly. Tell the child to feel the body first, heavy and comfortable, but then begin to lighten. At this point, I like to say "Bring this feeling of relaxation and comfort with you today, as far as you can take it." If the imagery helps a symptom such as a headache, then I add, "Take this freedom from pain [or diminished pain] with you into your day." A slow return works well: counting backwards from ten to one is a nice way to accomplish this return with your child. "One" is fully awake with eyes open. Do not let the child sit up quickly but, rather, in stages, slowly rising. Once the child is sitting up, offer a glass of clean, clear water. Drinking with water grounds the body, bringing it "back" and helping the child to be present.

In the grounding stage, let the child talk about the imagery and jot down notes if needed. This is also the time for the child to write or draw about his or her experience as well, making it familiar and more concrete. It is also a time for listening on the parent's part. I have found that the process remains active after the actual session, and that later in the day or week is when children draw, write, and continue to talk about the particular imagery. The imagery process is like the healing process; it is ongoing and active.

Imagery

"Aerodynamically, the bumblebee shouldn't be able to fly, but the bumblebee doesn't know it so it goes on flying anyway."

–Mary Kay Ash

The following imageries are written to help your child cope with particular symptoms. Some of these imageries are for overall wellness, while others are to be used for more specific symptoms, such as fever. They are written in story-like form and are adaptable to any personal touches you want to add. For example, you may want to add the use of your child's favorite color. Prior to reading imagery, it is recommended you do a relaxation exercise. Once both you and your child are relaxed, you can begin your imagery session.

The Healing Garden (Flu)

This imagery can be used for flu symptoms.
Do the relaxation exercise prior to this imagery.

You don't feel well at all. You ache all over, and this feeling makes you frightened and unhappy. You don't like to be sick and miss out on play-time. But you can make yourself feel better and stronger. Relax your body, shut your eyes, and take deep, slow breaths. Imagine a beautiful,

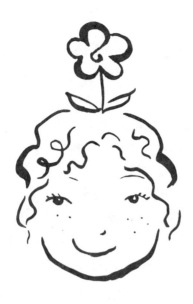

purple pouch tied with a golden ribbon. Open this magical pouch, and you see it is filled with shimmering seeds. They are all different shapes and sizes. Now imagine the inside of your body filled with soft, brown earth. It is perfect for planting, so go ahead and start to plant your seeds. Take handfuls of these healing seeds, and spread them all throughout your body. As you spread them, they light up your earth, and you start to feel better. The seeds sink into your warm, soft, inner garden and start to grow almost immediately. You secretly hope they are flower seeds. They start to sprout their little roots, and it tickles you inside. The seeds start to push their tiny sprouts out of your earth, and that tickles you too and makes you smile. Your heart is their sun, giving them warmth, light, and love. That is all a plant or a child needs to grow and get bigger and stronger! You can see the green of the sprouts and leaves, but you still don't know what they will become. Concentrate, and watch the plants grow and blossom into what you wished for—flowers! You see hundreds of beautiful, dazzling flowers filling your whole body. There are daisies, roses, dandelions, and tulips coming up everywhere, filling you with color. If you try hard, you can actually smell their lovely blossoms. Their colors and fragrances are powerful and healing. This power you can use to make yourself feel better. Your scared and sick feelings are leaving you now and you feel happy and healthy! Your special garden is for you and no one else. It is magnificent, healing, and wondrous, and you are lucky to have it.

Recall: Relax, take deep, slow breaths, and relax your body. Imagine your special garden with its soft, rich earth. You can open your magic pouch anytime, anyplace, and plant your seeds anytime, anyplace. Spread them, and watch your flowers grow and bring you strength and happiness. Their sweet smell and bright colors warm you and fill you with love, and you feel better. Relax, and watch them grow. Your garden is the most beautiful one in the world, and it lives in you!

The Fire Engines (Fever)

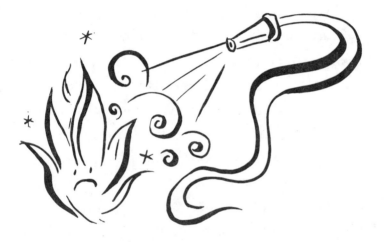

This imagery can be used for fever control.
Do the relaxation exercise prior to this imagery.

YOUR BODY is feeling warm, but not in a good way. It is uncomfortable for you, and you do not like it at all. You want to be cool and happy, but everything seems to be so hot. It's those horrible Flamies that are making you feel yucky all over. Giving a temperature to little children is their most favorite thing to do. Their bright yellow-orange color makes you feel as if your body is boiling inside. But you have the power to fight them. You really do, and all you have to do is believe.

Close your eyes lightly, relax, and start to take slow, deep breaths. Imagine a cool spray of clean, crystal-clear water. This special water has a healing power that will help you, but you say, "Where is it coming from?" Now you start to see movement in the distance, and it's a shiny, perfect red. Slowly you start to see something. . . . It's a hundred beautiful, red Fire Engines, and they are streaming into your body. They can enter through your nose, your mouth, and your ears. They have no taste, thank goodness! And they are very quiet, for now, because they do not have their sirens on. These mighty Fire Engines are also in your medicine, so be sure to take it! The Flamies don't like to see the Fire Engines coming, because they know the Fire Engines have something very powerful. As they fill your body, you start to feel better almost immediately. They are actually tickling and cooling your insides. They fill you up with their love and strength.

When the Fire Engines meet up with the Flamies, they blast them with their sirens to

Child

scare them. The Flamies fight back by blazing their hot, yellow color brighter. But the Fire Engines have big tanks on their backs, and they are full of lovely, cool water. This healing water is cleansing and magical. They raise their hoses at the burning Flamies, and a huge spray of cold luminous water hits a bunch of the Flamies—and they disappear! The Fire Engines race all over your body with their sirens going, chasing the Flamies and putting out their fires. You are cooling down now, but all their cold water sometimes makes you feel a chill. But you know that is okay, because you are already cool and comfortable. Your body feels good again. You are so happy to have friends like the red Fire Engines and their wonderful, powerful water.

Recall: Anytime you are feeling bad and think you may be getting a temperature, you can always make yourself feel better. Calm down and relax your body. Shut your eyes lightly, and take some deep, slow breaths. Now sound the secret fire alarm that only you and the Fire Engines can hear. They will come and help you anytime you call on them. They love you very much and are always there for you. They will always get rid of the hot Flamies with their cold, pure water. Now, imagine and bring them into your body and let them do what they love to do . . . put out the fire.

The Pink Kittens (Younger Child)
Dedicated to Libby.

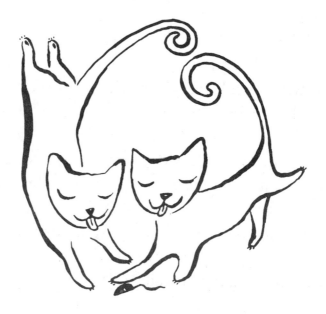

This imagery can be used for the younger child.
Do the relaxation exercise prior to this imagery.

FEELING SICK is no fun, no fun at all! You feel achy all over, and your tummy is upset. You're very afraid that you may have to throw up. Nobody likes to throw up, especially little kids. You try to stay quiet like your Mom or Dad [or caretaker] said, but you can't get comfortable. What is going on inside you, you wonder? What is being sick? It is all so hard to understand. You know that something is not right inside your body. You decide to call this feeling Mischief Mice. They scurry around inside you, and it makes you feel sick. These little gray creatures have red eyes and they scare you, and you want them to go away. But you can make them go away if you believe in magic!

Make believe you are going to take a little nap. You are going to relax your body and shut your eyes. Try not to wiggle! Now start to take deep, slow breaths like you do at the doctor's office. You can feel yourself relaxing and becoming quiet. Now picture your friends the pretty Pink Kittens. They are playing with each other when you call them, and then they stop and pick up their ears, listening. You call again, and they come running, tumbling all over each other, each trying to be first, like in a race. They are a little bit silly because they are just kittens, but very special—because they are PINK! Your Pink Kittens are so adorable and fluffy. You can actually feel their soft, pink fur inside you, and it tickles! But the best part is that they are magical and have the power to make you feel better, just like your medicine. You know where their magic comes from? Their little pink tongues! You tell them you want to feel better, and they start to chase happily after the Mischief Mice. When your Pink Kittens catch them, they lick each one, and each and every Mischief Mouse disappears! Your special friends, the Pink Kittens, are all over your body, making it feel good again. All the mean mice are gone. You are feeling well again, and you love your Pink Kittens very much. And they love you too!

Recall: Anytime you don't feel well or are scared, you can call your special friends, the Pink Kittens, to help you. Shut your eyes, and relax your body, taking slow, deep breaths. Now call to your Pink Kittens and have them visit your body. Only you and your Pink Kittens can hear you call them. You Pink Kittens know that the Mischief Mice make you feel bad. Tell them what you need. Tell them to go lick away those pesky Mischief Mice and make them disappear. They will do anything for you. You love to watch them playing and racing after the mice. It makes you feel happy inside to have them to help you when you need them.

YOUR MAGIC PAINT BOX (PAIN)

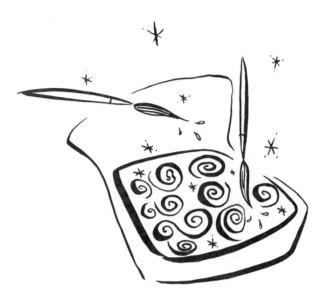

This imagery can be used for pain control.
Do the relaxation exercise prior to this imagery.

IN YOUR SPECIAL PAINT BOX, you have more colors than anyone else in the world. There is the lightest, purest white to the darkest, deepest black, and everything else in between. Healing purple, lovely pink, sunny yellow, and blissful blue. Imagine every color and hue of a tremendous rainbow within your paint box. Being the largest paint box in the world, it also has the largest paint brushes! These marvelous brushes have the softest bristles and make the biggest and best strokes. You love your paint box and all of its beautiful, powerful colors. It is a good thing you have this wonderful paint box because it is magical and can help make you feel better whenever you have pain or if you're unhappy in some way.

When you get hurt or have pain, the Nasties appear. When you are feeling pain or when you are weak and scared, they are very cruel and love to make little children go to their beds so they have to miss school and all the fun with friends. Of course, the Nasties are an awful color. They are a creepy gray-green that looks mean and painful. And they have no real shape; they are just messy blobs. But they can be powerful and can make you hurt, if you let them. But you have much more power within you, and you have a way to fight them. All you have to do is imagine and try. Stay relaxed. It makes you stronger. Concentrate and picture your wonderful paint box in your mind. Slowly open the cover of your huge paint box, and watch the magnificent paint brushes work their magic. These brushes fill their bristles with thick, rich paint. They enter your body at the top of your head, slowly filling you with love, and painting rainbows all the way down to your toes. When they meet the ugly, painful Nasties inside your body, they brush each one with the powerful, healing colors, and the pain goes away! When each Nasty is touched by the paint brushes, it becomes the dazzling color of the paint it was touched with, and all the meanness and power go away! As the colors spread, the Nasties disappear, and so does your pain and fear. You are filled with an enormous rainbow that is mighty and healing, a rainbow that makes you happy, feeling healthy, pain-free, and loved.

Recall: Whenever you hurt and have pain, ask your magic paint box to help you, anytime, anyplace. Shut your eyes, relax your body, and take some slow, deep breaths. Picture opening up your paint box. No one else has to know what you're dreaming of. Let the colorful, healing paint brushes enter, in a small stream, through the top of your head again. Fill your body with the splendid colors of your own splendid rainbow, replacing the pain with all the colors of the rainbow. Now let them do their job, and paint away the Nasties. Ahhh . . . it feels so good!

The Fairy Bubbles (Breathing)

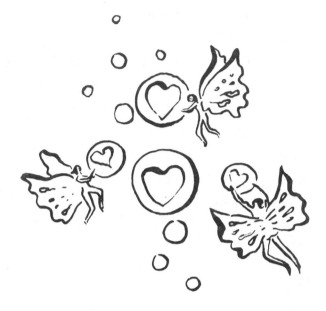

This imagery can be used for difficulty breathing.
Do the relaxation exercise prior to this imagery.

Whenever you start to have that feeling—you know, when you start to feel your chest tighten or the nasty cough starts, or both!—you have the power, with the help of the Fairy Bubbles, to stop this feeling and breathe perfectly. Inside your body, the mean cells, called the Wheezies, love to make your lungs go crazy. They are happy when they wreck your day or wake you up in the middle of the night, making it hard for you to breathe and scaring you. These

Wheezies are shaped like small nets, made out of elastic and mucus (kind of like boogies). They wrap themselves around the tubes in your lungs, even the tiny ones, and squeeze. That's why you can't take a deep breath.

But you can fight them if you believe you can. Relax your body, and sit any way you like. Just be comfortable. Imagine the tiniest fairies on the earth. There are boy fairies and girl fairies of every color you can imagine. They have shiny, silver wings that make a lovely, pleasant humming sound. Each one of them is carrying a delicate, silver bubble. They are your magical friends who can help you breathe. They really can. The silver bubbles are called Fairy Bubbles, and they are filled with magic, medicine, and healing love. The fairies enter your body through your mouth and quickly fly to your lungs. There are millions of them inside of you! Now they let go of their magical Fairy Bubbles—and the Fairy Bubbles burst and send a spray of the most powerful breathing medicine in the world, into your lungs! All the Wheezies' nets break and vanish. Your whole chest opens up immediately, and you can breath again. The Fairy Bubbles are everywhere, in your lungs, throat, mouth, and nose. You are calming down, and the wheezing and tightness is going away. Your wonderful, happy fairies are laughing and playing, and they are so pleased that you chose them to help you. You are happy, too, because now you know you have your special magical friends to help you whenever you need them. They leave your body now, to rest and make more bubbles for you, back in Fairyland. The fairies and their Fairy Bubbles will come back anytime, anyplace. Just believe, and you have the power to make it happen!

Recall: Whenever you start to wheeze or cough and you think you are starting to have a asthma attack, there is something you can do, while you take your medicine. Relax your body and take slow, deep breaths. Now call your special fairy friends. You can start to hear a lovely humming sound, and you know they are on their way. The tiny fairies want to come and help you. They are carrying their silver Fairy Bubbles and flying right into your lungs. The bubbles are bursting all over the place and the tubes in your lungs are opening! You can breathe again, and the scared feeling is leaving you. Your beautiful, tiny fairies have done another good job! You love them, and they love you, too. They will come to help you any time you need them.

THE DEER FAMILY (SLEEP)

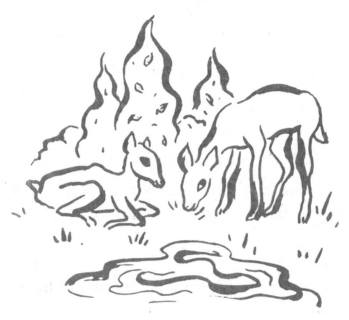

*This imagery can be used for sleep problems.
Do the relaxation exercise prior to this imagery.*

ONCE you are comfortable and relaxed, imagine a beautiful summer afternoon. You are looking at the gentle swaying of a field of grass in a large, safe meadow. There are flowers scattered throughout the meadow, and you can smell their wonderful scent on the wind. There are birds calling to each other over the rustling trees that surround the meadow. The wind is warm and soft on your face. As you stand there, take in all the sights and sounds of this place.

You're happy you are there. As you stand in the meadow, you see something stir at an opening in the wood. Curious, you begin to walk toward the opening, and you find a small path in a pine grove.

You enter along the path quietly, walking out of the sunshine to the cool shade of the wood. The scent of pine and earth meets your nose in a burst. Your eyes take a moment to adjust, and you see your path clearly again. There is another stirring in front of you, so you go on. The path curls around the trees and leads to a clear, cool stream. You can hear and smell the stream before you see it. As you come out of the woods, you come face to face with the most beautiful mother deer, drinking at the stream. You stop and smile, and she stays halfway in the stream, looking directly into your eyes. She seems to be smiling too. You slowly walk toward her, and she actually lets you stroke her strong head and shoulders. She nestles up against you for a moment. You are feeling so happy and thrilled that a real deer is letting you touch her! She is soft as silk, and her fur is sleek. She takes one last drink and turns slowly, crossing the stream.

She waits for you on the other side. She wants you to follow her. You wade through the cool water and follow her into the other side of the cool, piney forest. Again it is cool and shady under the trees. You round a large bush and, to your surprise, there is a fawn curled up on the warm, soft grass under the bush. The fawn lifts its head, and you look into the deepest, most beautiful eyes you have ever seen. You smile at the fawn's mother and she nods her head yes, letting you go nearer to her baby. You sit down, and you smell the soft, natural, woody scent of the fawn. You quietly pat the fawn, whispering sweet words of love to him. As you do this there is a sound from the woods, a heavy step. The father deer, in all his glory, has arrived. He is magnificent, the king of the woods. He has very large antlers and is twice the size of his wife. He looks from you to his baby and then to his wife. He seems to relax a bit and nuzzles the fawn, brushing your hand with his warm lips. Then he and his wife head off into the woods, leaving you with the baby. They trust you to take care of him! As they disappear, you notice that your body has suddenly become very tired. The baby deer puts his head down and goes to sleep. You curl up against the warm sweet fawn. You breathe in his soft smell of sweet grass, pine, and tender fur. Now you are very tired too. You slowly drift into a deep sleep, knowing you are safe with your friends, the deer.

Recall: If you are feeling tired and tense you can always go to see your beautiful deer friends. Relax and take slow, deep breaths, relaxing. Slowing down and releasing any tension you may be holding in your body. You start to hear the whisper of your wonderful stream and the delicate scent of the forest's pine trees. It is quiet and peaceful in this place. You call for your deer family members. You can see them slowly walking towards you. You feel calmer and sleepier just seeing them. Reach out and call to them. Let them come to you and rest with you. You nuzzle up to the baby deer again smelling its warm fur. The baby deer licks your hands and you are even more calm and quiet. Rest and be happy knowing your deer family is always with you when you need them. Good night and sleep well.

YOUR POWERFUL SOCCER TEAM (FEAR)

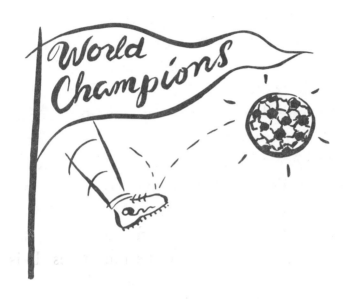

This imagery can be used for fear.
Do the relaxation exercise prior to this imagery.

YOU are very lucky because you have your own special soccer team! They are extra special because they have the power and magic to make you feel strong and brave. You are the coach and the owner, all rolled up in one, so you are totally in charge of this championship team! You can make their uniforms any color you like and call them any name you wish. Your Powerful Soccer Team is undefeated when it comes to making kids feel powerful. All the soccer players are huge, powerful, and World Champions. They believe in making kids feel better and will play any team to meet that goal. (Now pick your team colors and name if you like.)

When you are scared, there is a wicked, raggedy soccer team, which can form inside your body. This soccer team is made up of all the rejects that could not make it in international soccer. Their uniforms and shoes are so dirty and old that you can't figure out what color they are. They do not care about anybody but themselves, and they certainly don't care about sick children! They are mean and mad when they get inside your body, and they refuse to follow the rules of the game. They cheat, get many penalties, and injure you or any other players they can. When they are inside your body you feel scared and unhappy. They like it when you can't play with your friends and have to stay in bed. But with the help and love from your Powerful Soccer Team, you can beat them easily.

Relax your body, shut your eyes, and take deep breaths, slowly. As your body calms itself, you hear the game whistle and see your team take the field. Each of your teammates looks magnificent. They are in top condition, and every muscle is perfect. They are determined to get rid of the evil, cheating team that robs you of your strength. You are feeling their strength and bravery. The game begins. Your powerful players frighten the other team! Each time one of your magical soccer players kicks the ball, an opponent disappears. Each time your team gets a goal, bunches of them disappear, magically! As the mean soccer players disappear, so do your frightened feelings. You see your special team celebrating and giving each other high fives because they are happy when they help a child like you win the game. You are not afraid anymore! In a very short time, they have taken over the field and have crushed the evil team—and, along with it, your lonely, scary feelings!

Recall: You can call your special soccer team whenever you need them. Sound a secret game whistle inside your body, a whistle that only you and the soccer players can hear. They will come when you call. They will help you feel stronger and get rid of the other harmful soccer team players who make you afraid and unhappy. The game is always swift and predictable. Goal after goal, you and your champions will always win the game! You have the power.

YOUR SPECIAL WEATHER REPORT (SIDE EFFECTS)

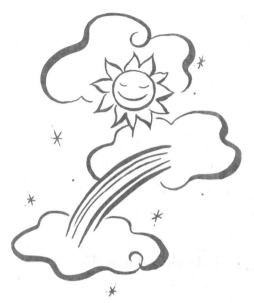

This imagery can be used for side effects.
Do the relaxation exercise prior to this imagery.

THERE IS A STORM BREWING inside your body, making you feel like you cannot breathe or eat or play. It is confusing to feel this way, especially for kids. Your weather report is not good; there is a storm warning. You can feel the dark, gloomy clouds forming inside your-body (this can happen after you have your medicine/chemotherapy). You feel the gray rain falling, with spikes of lightning and loud claps of thunder, making you feel scared. But you can change your weather report and feel better, if you try! All you have to do is believe you can!

Relax your whole body. Start to take slow, deep breaths with your eyes shut. Watch the rain and imagine it changing into big drops of brilliant diamonds. These healing diamonds are precious and valuable because they make you well again. Imagine the storm clouds slowly turning from their dark, scary color to a powdery, wispy white. Your feelings of discomfort are going away. The lightning is changing too. Instead of jagged, sharp shapes, it is softening, curling, and slowing down. Everything is slowing down. It is drifting and curling into your body, making you relax. You feel restored. The lightning still has its powerful energy, but now it is helping you, instead of hurting you or making you feel sick. Your bad weather is moving out and making way for good weather.

Your glorious sun is starting to shine, and its warmth overflows within you. The air smells clean and healing. You do not feel bad anymore! The sky is a bright blue with a few puffy, white clouds. A stunning rainbow forms, and its broad, smiling face beams down on you. It fills you with love and makes you feel much better and happier. All your bad symptoms are melting away. You have made the storm inside you go away. You brought the cheerful, good weather back, just by believing! You take a big breath. It is clear and quiet, and it gives you no fear.

Recall: Whenever you feel a storm brewing inside you and you want it to go away, all you have to do is believe—and it can happen! Relax your body and shut your eyes softly. Take slow, deep breaths, and imagine moving the stormy weather out of your body. Bring in your dazzling rain diamonds and your healing lightning. Let them get rid of any sick feelings you have. The rain clouds disappear. The brilliant sunshine and your big, bold rainbow are left. You and you alone know when you have to call your special weather friends to help you. They will come and take the bad weather away, anytime, anyplace. Believe, and it will come true.

YOUR NIGHTTIME FRIENDS (COPING)

This imagery can be used for general symptoms.
Do the relaxation exercise prior to this imagery.

IMAGINE the most beautiful, midnight-blue sky above you. It is absolutely jam-packed with

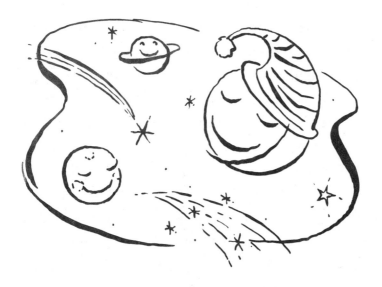

radiant stars, spinning planets, and, of course, the brilliant moon. You can see the entire galaxy shining over you. The Milky Way is a dazzling nighttime pathway ready to help heal you. These special Nighttime Friends are always ready for you when you feel sick or unhappy. They will help you feel all better, just like when you take your medicine. All you have to do is believe!

Inside your body there are shadows that make you feel tired, sick, and unable to play. These shadows are tiny but very troublesome, especially for kids. They are very mean because they love to make you cry, and you get scared when you feel this way. But thank goodness there is a way to fight them. Your beautiful stars, planets, and moon will rescue you! The wondrous Milky Way has more strength than any power the shadows may have.

Relax, and breathe slowly and deeply. Shut your eyes, and imagine the midnight-blue sky in your mind. The shiny stars and planets stream into your body through the top of your head and fill you to the tips of your toes. Now pull the powerful Milky Way down and into your body. You are starting to feel restored and better already. The moon shines down on you, and your body is brimming over with its light. The shadows hate the light. Your sparkling Nighttime Friends flow to all parts of your body and destroy the shadows with their golden beams. The planets rocket into your body and hit a large shadow with all their might. There is an explosion of light all over your body; it's the Milky Way coming to your rescue! The ever-present moon smiles and radiates its constant, steady happiness down onto you. The shadows have gone because of your powerful light, and you are feeling healthier, happier, and strong. You are lucky to have such special Nighttime Friends.

Child

Recall: Whenever you are starting to feel sick or scared, you can have your special Nighttime Friends come into your body, even during the day! Just shut your eyes, breathe slowly and deeply, and relax your body. Think of that sparkling, midnight-blue sky with the stars shining, the planets moving, and the moon smiling. Let their healing energy enter through the top of your head once again. They love to visit and help you with their shine and their glow, especially the giant Milky Way! They dissolve all the shadows with their celestial light. As the last shadow vanishes, you are well again, feeling happy and safe. You are overflowing with the healing light of your special Nighttime Friends.

THE MAGICAL MUSICAL NOTES (WOUND HEALING)

This imagery can be used for injury.
Do the relaxation exercise prior to this imagery.

RELAX your body, shut your eyes, and take deep, slow breaths. Quiet your body inside and out. Now imagine the sound of the most beautiful music you have ever heard. It is the sound of happiness, love, and magic—all rolled into one.

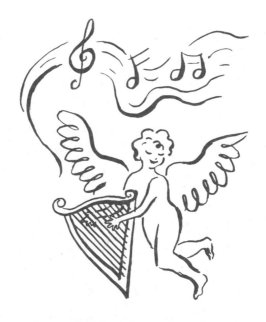

It sounds light and peaceful as you just relax and listen. Your body needs the nourishment from this healing sound, especially where you hurt yourself [broken bone, laceration]. You imagine a big symphony orchestra in your mind, but, to your surprise, it turns out to be not an orchestra at all. It is thousands of angels playing their radiant, golden harps. You can see the little black musical notes fly from the harps every time angels stroke their fingers across the strings. These little black notes carry goodness and healing power in each one of them and can help to heal your hurt [_____]. And who could be better than an angel to deliver these healing notes to your body?!

Child

You have been injured and have hurt your [_____]. It has been very frightening and painful for you. But now you need to heal, and your body needs the sound of healing. This sound of healing and beautiful music will come from your angels. With the help of your angels' music and your medicine, you can help yourself. You can decrease your pain and heal your [_____]. Just believe, and it can happen!

Your golden angels enter your body through your ears and make you glow inside. Listen to them play their harps, making their special magical music. All of the beautiful musical notes jump from the brilliant harps, spreading their healing sounds throughout your body. The minute your body starts to hear the wonderful sounds, it feels better, and the discomfort you have in your [_____] is disappearing. Let these bad feelings melt away, each note entering and healing. You are starting to feel much better, much stronger, and much happier. Listen to your lovely angels making the most gorgeous music you have ever heard. Imagine the musical notes strengthening your cells and making your body mend itself. The powerful, healing musical notes are overflowing in all parts of your body. As the music plays, you are becoming stronger, happier, and full of love. All you have to do is believe. Watch your friends, the angels, and listen to their healing music.

Recall: Know that anytime you want, you can bring the magical music into your body to help heal your [_____]. Just relax, shut your eyes lightly and breathe deeply and slowly. Imagine these heavenly angels entering your body. Silently ask them to play their elegant harps for you, sending out their healing sounds. Only you and your angels can hear the music. As the music begins, you can feel the warm glow again inside your body. As the magical notes sound throughout your body, you can feel your pain melting away. Play your internal music, and let your body heal. Make yourself well again.

How to Create Your Own Imagery

"WHAT WOULD YOU ATTEMPT TO DO IF YOU KNEW YOU WOULD NOT FAIL?"

–Robert Schuller

THE EXPERIENCE of imagery has jumpstarted several different inner workings in your child, as well as in yourself. We have discussed imagination, trust, honor, and teamwork as parts of the imagery process. Taking these ingredients, with a little imagination and creativity, you as a parent-child team can create your own personalized and unique imagery. You have to leave your "I can't" behind and change it to "I can" or at least "I will try." This may be more difficult for you than for your child, but just following the child's lead is the best advice. As you have discovered with imagery, children's minds are fertile gardens, ready to grow and flower. Creating their own imagery is a natural step for children after learning the overall imagery process. Writing your own imagery stories together can make the entire experience extremely meaningful for both child and parent, because the imagery is grounded in personal experience. Adding personal information, such as the name of the child's medication, type of procedure, or names of important team members, can help the child identify with the imagery more strongly. For example, if your teen or child is a diabetic and you have incorporated imagery into the overall wellness plan, then bring the words *syringe, diet,* or *insulin* into your imagery story. If your child has to endure a difficult procedure, use the words *catheter, medication,* or *intravenous fluid* in your imagery stories. It will make it more comfortable for both of you. Navigating in more familiar waters with terms that have particular meaning for your child's needs and situation strengthens the imagery story. Also remember the power of touch. Incorporate it into your child's imagery at any point. You can tape your imagery stories, bringing the experience full circle. This tape becomes your special creation as parent and child. Building a story and identifying important familiar names and situations help the child, once again, to be part of the process. And as a parent you can re-experience the benefits of "letting go" of control and of trusting the process.

When the recipe calls for fantasy, color, or beings with a good measurement of imagination, your child can cook up a magical, empowering story, blending reality with fun. The delight for the child is in taking all the ingredients that make your child special and creating imagery that will continue to teach, expand, and heal. So just add all these ingredients and stir.

The following is an example to further help you in creating your own unique imagery. Using the image of a lighthouse as a symbol of guidance and light, you can create an imagery that can help any symptom or situation your child may be experiencing. In guided directed imagery, after a relaxation exercise has been done, help the child bring forth an image of a lighthouse. Then further assist the child in imagining a heavy load or burden (which represents a symptom). As the child ascends the lighthouse steps, let each step lighten the load, shedding the weight and burden. If you are using a specific symptom, have the child decrease that unwanted symptom while ascending the stairs to the top of the lighthouse. You can create the goal of being symptom free by the time the pinnacle of the lighthouse is reached. You can extend further into the imagery by having the child

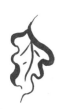

know that the lighthouse's light and power are within. The combinations in this imagery alone are endless.

In Interactive Guided Imagery[SM], the child interacts with personal images, but you as guide can still help the child bring this shedding of a burden to the interactive imagery technique. Just trust the process, all of it. Listen, and use your imagination. The rest is all about love.

Five: *Interactive Guided Imagery*^{SM}

"WE ARE UPLIFTED BY NATURAL BEAUTY, BECAUSE OUR
OWN INNER NATURE RESPONDS."
                    -Joan Goldstein and Manuela Soares,
                            authors of The Joy Within

INTERACTIVE GUIDED IMAGERY^{SM} and Interactive
Imagery^{SM} are service marked terms that represent a particular form of guided imagery developed and taught by
the Academy for Guided Imagery. Located in Mill
Valley, California, the Academy trains and certifies health
professionals in the Interactive Guided Imagery^{SM}
approach and provides resources for the public. In this
form of guided imagery, the child or teenager actually
learns to interface with the mind's images to become
more aware of many unconscious health issues and problems, including symptoms. This more in-depth technique
takes imagery one step further. It can assist children in
discovering their own unique healing images or pictures
and then guide them in a process of interacting with
those images in a kind of inner dialogue. This inner dialogue often results in unusually powerful experiences that
are long remembered. Working with images in this way
enables a child to explore and bring fresh insight and
understanding to medical problems and symptoms, both
minor and severe, listening to the small voice within.

The many different imagery techniques taught in
this chapter—such as pain control imagery, evocative

imagery, conflict resolution, and the use of recall—are techniques developed and taught by the Academy of Guided Imagery in their imagery training. If you learn these different techniques, you will have a well-stocked "toolbag" to help your child in a time of need. Ultimately, you will see how to use multiple interactive techniques in much greater detail.

Imagery works. Trust the process. Naturally, with practice you will discover what is appropriate and comfortable for you and your child. I have found that using a combination of techniques works nicely with children. Whether you read guided imagery, or work with images directly, the child will learn the gift of self-healing.

An important point to remember is always to do a relaxation of some kind prior to doing a session, whether it is guided imagery or Interactive Guided Imagery^{SM}. The relaxation can be simple and short, or elaborate and long, whatever you and yours prefer.

Interactive Guided Imagery^{SM} is used in private practitioners' offices, connected both with mental health and with medical specialties. It is being used increasingly in the hospital setting for pre-operative and post-operative care. It is used for minor and major procedures, with positive results. Interactive Imagery^{SM} is a very powerful self-healing process. The following are some of the ways Interactive Guided Imagery^{SM} has been used in many clinical and home settings.

- Relaxing and reducing stress
- Reducing anxiety
- Relieving pain and symptoms

- Preparing for surgery
- Potentiating the action of medications and treatments
- Minimizing side effects
- Dealing with chronic illness
- Empowering the patient
- Tolerating difficult procedures
- Preparing for labor and delivery
- Accessing inner wisdom and guidance
- Accessing insights and information concerning a particular problem or situation
- Actively participating in the healing process
- Addressing emotional expression or release
- Exploring/understanding parts and aspects of the self
- Finding meaning in illness/crisis
- Enhancing coping skills

Interactive Imagery^{SM} Techniques

"THE GREATEST REVOLUTION OF OUR GENERATION IS THE DISCOVERY THAT HUMAN BEINGS, BY CHANGING THE INNER ATTITUDES OF THEIR MINDS, CAN CHANGE THE OUTER ASPECTS OF THEIR LIVES."

-*William James*

The Special Place

ONE OF MY ALL TIME FAVORITES, the "special place" imagery! What could be better than to feel as if you can go somewhere new, filled with beauty and safety—and you can go there anytime you wish? That is basically how the special place works. Once relaxed, the child can be guided to a special place, real or imagined. It is a personal, private place of beauty, healing, and peace. It can be anything the child wants—a tropical beach, the top of a mountain, or maybe the simplicity of his or her own bedroom. You use sensory recruitment to initiate and maintain the imagery, directing or guiding the child when guidance is needed (e.g., "What do you hear?" "What type of weather is it?"). Be patient and open. The image will come. Each time you and your child do the special place imagery, the place can change or stay the same. Most kids stick to one place for awhile and then get a bit bored and want to "go on to a new place." Then they usually have a number of special places to go. One of the written imageries in this book is The Trekking Dial (p. 148), which is a directive form of imagery that invites the teen or older child to go to many exotic and beautiful places.

Using the special place as a starting point in both guided imagery and Interactive Imagery^SM is very helpful and effective. I believe the reason for this effectiveness is because it is easy to do (for most) because of the "getting away" factor. When sick or hurt, children or adults many times "just want to get away," whether that means away from the symptoms, the procedures, the discomfort, or the stress. These feelings can result in more harmful reactions such as frustration and anger. But with relaxation and imagery, getting away for even a moment is possible! Much like the "minis," the special place can be recalled, benefiting that child or teen at that moment. After the parent initiates relaxation, the special place imagery can begin.

I have been able to teach many children to do "recall" with their eyes open. This works well in certain situations, such as when the child or teen is at school and experiencing symptoms of discomfort. I do advise that the teachers and school nurse know that the child does this "self biofeedback" technique so that there will be no misunderstandings. Of course, the most common way to relax and do imagery is with the eyes closed, but there are situations when the child may not want to do this. It is a technique that takes a little practice, but it can be done. For the quick "recall" type of imagery, the child can find a focal point and start to take some slow, deep breaths. There is a certain amount of zoning out of the surrounding sounds. The child can then bring forth an image of a pain scale and work the pain down in intensity, or speak to the inner advisor for support and advice (refer to p. 112). All the while, the eyes are open, and the child is still somewhat "present." It is a form of daydreaming, but it is much more directed to accomplishing a certain outcome. It all takes about a minute, but can improve the situation quickly and positively. Many youths I have worked with use this technique as well as the "longer" imagery, in the school nurse's office when the technique is needed. Instead of going home from school, they are able to reduce their symptoms and finish the school day.

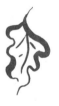

*Please note: The words in brackets are ongoing cues for parents
while guiding the child during imagery.
Do a relaxation exercise prior to this imagery.*

Take quiet, deep breaths ... relax your body
... make yourself quiet and calm ... let go of any
tension ... deep breathing ... listen to your
breath.... Now that you are relaxed and quiet
... bring forth an image of a beautiful, peaceful,
safe place ... it can be anywhere you want ... it
can be anywhere at all. Just let it form. This
place is filled with healing and quiet ... it is for
you and for you alone.... When you are ready,
raise a finger (nod your head) to let me know
when you are there. [This is where the child is
interacting with the image and giving you information during that interacting.] Good [slowly]
... what are you seeing? What are you hearing?
Do you smell anything? [Be patient, and give
time for the child to do the work. Nothing
should be rushed.] What time of day is it? What
is the weather? ... tell me more ... [Encourage
communication with the image.] Take a
moment to sit in your special place and take in
all its beauty, healing, safety, and quiet ... let me
know if anything changes ... enjoy your special
place. It is yours and yours alone ... you can
come here anytime you wish. When you are

ready, begin to return to the room...taking your time ... thinking of your breathing again ... hearing the sounds in the room ... slowly ... begin opening your eyes ... your body relaxed, comfortable. You are refreshed from your visit to your special place.

As discussed previously, it is very important to the imagery experience to do a wrap-up and assessment following the session. Expressing feelings after the imagery is a wonderful release for the child and can bring added insight to the process.

Wrap-up: Let the child tell you about the experience of the special place and how it felt. Ask questions: Did anything surprise you? Did your feelings change from the start of the session to the ending of the session? Did you learn anything new today?

If the introduction of the special place for any reason seems to be impossible for the child or teenager to image, don't push it. Sadly, there are some children who do not have any place that feels safe, even in their own minds and hearts. If the child becomes frightened or tense, or starts to cry, it is time to stop the imagery, which can be done by having the child open the eyes and return to the room slowly. Do not let the child get up quickly, because it can sometimes cause dizziness.

This situation may require a hug and some reassurance. The child does not have to do the special place imagery as the starting point. Together you can pick another way to begin the imagery session. I think it is also appropriate to explore the child's lack of feeling safe with a professional.

The Inner Advisor/Healer

THIS IMAGERY is number two on my list of hits, the fascinating technique of the "Inner Advisor." The parent guides the child to bring forth an image that represents wisdom, love, support, and safety. This image can be anything: a family member, an animal, a spiritual figure, a shape, or even a presence. Inner advisors can be guardian angels, imaginary friends, or simple intuition—that important small voice within. The child is guided to interact with that image while the parent aids the child in describing the image and asking the image questions. Keep in mind that listening is an important part of the parent's role. Be patient, and give time for the child to do the work. It is essential that nothing should be rushed, and patience on the parent's part is vital. When the child or teen is interacting with the imagery, it is an active process. The inner advisor is the liaison between the conscious and the subconscious mind and is a powerful concept and tool. In imagery, the guidance from the inner advisor figure makes our unconscious minds more accessible. The inner advisor is a wonderful image for the child to interact with because many times the advisor has the answers to the child's feelings about specific symptoms. The inner advisor figure can be used for support, diagnosis, conflict resolution, problem-solving, and symptom control. Martin Rossman, M.D., of the Academy of Guided Imagery has said, "[Y]our whole inner mind is an advisor because it contains a vast amount of information about you and your well-being. It will naturally try to express those thoughts, feelings, and actions that are most important in your life. When you ask your image about something, whether it's a symptom, an illness, a problem, or a feeling, the image will give you information about that 'something' which you may not have been aware of." [7]

Another way to think of it is to ask the question: "Who knows you better than you do?" You actually have all the answers to the questions that concern yourself, but they are deep inside under many layers. This pertains to a child as well as an adult, but the child just may not be sophisticated enough to have the tools to get answers to those deeper questions. The inner healer or advisor gives the child these tools. It is an image of a person or thing that is more concrete (though built in the imagination) to work with. Keep in mind that the image can speak to the child with words or telepathically. For a kinetic child, the inner advisor may be a feeling or a presence. Through the senses, this imagined image helps the child to touch the inner core or being, with awakened and heightened awareness in order to be able to listen to the small voice within. This connection is especially crucial concerning health issues. Naturally, a young child may not immediately grasp how the inner advisor works, and that's okay. The parent should not get hung up on a lot of explaining to the child, so let the process take its course. Keep in mind that you can use a different word instead of *advisor* or *healer*. I have used *doctor*, *helper*, *friend*, or *nurse*, usually in the case of a younger child.

Inner advisors can help with all aspects of exploration in imagery. They are there for guidance and advice, assisting in answering questions about symptoms, diagnosis, and treatment. They help the children and teens to uncover information, solve problems, and resolve conflict.

Do a relaxation exercise prior to the imagery.

You are taking quiet, deep breaths ... relaxing your body ... making yourself quiet and calm ... letting go of any tension ... deeply breathing ... listening to your breath.... Now that you are relaxed and quiet ... feeling open and comfortable ... go to your special place and let an image ... or picture come to you.... This image is very nice and would never hurt you. It is here to help you ... it can be anything at all ... a person ... an animal ... just let it form.... It is someone or something that is safe and very wise ... just let it come ... it will answer any questions you may have ... take your time ... there is no rush ... slowly.... When you are ready, raise a finger (nod your head) to let me know you are ready.... When this image comes to you, take a moment to become relaxed and comfortable with it, looking at it. [This is where the child is interacting with the image and giving you information during that interaction.] Go slowly ... What does it look like? ... Tell me more ... go ahead and introduce yourself, and ask the image its name ... ask your advisor if it is going to help you ... letting the image talk to you ... answer you ... [Encourage communication with the image.] ... no rush ... ask the image any question you may have today ... anything about your illness (symptoms). What does it say? ... Tell me more ... [Be patient and give time for the child to do the work. Nothing should be rushed.] If this image cannot help you, ask if there is someone or something else that could. If so, ask the image to introduce you to this "new" image. [Repeat the above questions to this image. It may be the true inner healer.] When you are finished, thank your new friend and advisor for coming today and answering your questions.... Offer a gift of thanks (e.g., berries if the image is a bird). Ask your advisor if it will meet with you again and continue to be there for you ...

When you are ready, begin to return to the room ... taking your time ... thinking of your breathing again ... hearing the sounds in the room ... slowly ... begin opening your eyes ... your body relaxed, comfortable ... feeling wonderful that you have a special friend(s) to help you whenever you need advice.

Wrap-up: Let the child tell you about the image of the inner advisor and how that felt. What did the child find out? Was anything about the imagery surprising? Did the inner advisor help? Did the feelings change from the start of the session to the end of the session? Did the child learn anything new?

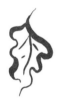

Please note that a child can have more than one inner advisor. Frequently, I have found that the first image may not be the true inner advisor/healer but, rather, a guide that introduces the child or teen to other images. I practice with some children who have numerous inner advisors to help them with specific issues. For one of my patients, there is "Stanley" the horse, for when the child feels the need for control and strength. There is "Dr. Chirp," the goldfinch who helps with all the little stomachaches and headaches. There is "Goldy" the fish who helps with math—and all the while "Lauren" the raccoon is the hostess, introducing new helpers that

live in the child's mind. As you can see, once the child
has started to trust imagery, the imagery can expand and
grow into many areas, helping the child in ways you
have never imagined.

Understanding an Image

AN IMAGE carries with it an immense amount of
emotional energy and brings the child or teen to a
deeper, better understanding of a particular situation,
need, or issue with special insight concerning symptoms. As a family, you have already gone through the
medical model and have an intimate knowledge of your
child's disease process and symptoms. You know them
not as the health care provider does, but as the parent—
and there is a difference. Imagery can enhance the
next level of your personal understanding of a symptom
or illness—by actually interacting with those symptoms or the illness.

This exploration of symptoms by the child or teen
can be met with some resistance, fear, or anxiety, because
the symptom has been a negative experience. Symptoms
are frightening and may have produced pain (emotional
or physical), so it is perfectly natural for the child to
resist. But expression of those feelings, as well as getting
a better understanding of them, is the positive outcome
to this particular exploratory imagery technique. The
parent as guide stimulates the child to use the senses to
bring the information through imagery. With gentle
guidance, the child is able to hear, feel, see, touch, and
even taste during the imagery. This sensory involvement

makes the process feel real, therefore producing real changes in the mind and then in the body.

There is new research emerging that shows some strong evidence that our cells have memory. Candace Pert, Ph.D., visiting professor at the Center for Molecular and Behavioral Neuroscience, Rutgers University (and former Chief of the Section on Brain Biochemistry of the Clinical Neuroscience Branch at the National Institute of Mental Health), states that "the immune system, like the central nervous system, has a memory and the capacity to learn. Thus it could be said that intelligence is located in literally every cell of the body, and that the traditional separation of mind and body no longer applies."[8]

Life events are linked to mental images, fused with the body itself, in the subconscious. Imagery links these two worlds. This integration is why imagery can teach children to self-heal and enhance overall wellness in mind, body, and spirit.

Do a relaxation exercise prior to this imagery.

You are taking quiet, deep breaths. . . . relaxing your body . . . making yourself quiet and calm . . . letting go of any tension . . . deeply breathing . . . listening to your breath. . . . Once you are relaxed and comfortable, let an image form, representing a symptom or problem that has been bothering you . . . no rush . . . go slowly . . . let the image form. It can be anything at all.

It can be any discomfort you are having...physically or emotionally. [Use the words about the body or emotions for the younger child.] Once it is there, observe it ... when you are ready, describe it. Does it have a shape, or color? What feelings does it make you have? Does this image have anything to say to you? What? Do you want to ask it a question? Do you want to tell this image anything? ... tell me more ... What are your feelings about it? You can be honest and tell it your true feelings...it's okay. [Encourage communication with the image.] Allow the image to answer you...what does it say? Will it work with you? Can you plan to meet with it again?...When you are ready, begin to return to the room ... take your time ... think of your breathing again ... you can hear the sounds in the room ... slowly ... begin opening your eyes ... your body is relaxed, comfortable. You feel good that you were able to be with this image and learn something from it.

Wrap-up: Ask questions: How do you feel? What have you learned? Did anything surprise you about this imagery? What does the image mean to you? Did your feelings change from the start of the session to the end of the session?

What will you do with this image? Did you learn anything new today?

Always let the child or teen know the advice an image gives doesn't have to be accepted. An example would be an inner advisor telling a teen to move out of the family home. Though this might come up as an answer from the image, the parent and teen need to discuss after the session the reasons this advice may not be a good option for the situation. Further exploration of the feelings behind this suggestion would be appropriate. One of your goals is to preserve the imagery process as a positive experience.

Pain Control

PAIN is a common symptom of many diseases. It can also be a difficult part of the treatment for a certain disease or injury. Many procedures and medications produce pain. It is one of the hardest symptoms for a child to endure and for a parent to witness. Both parent and child can feel totally helpless in this situation if pain gets the upper hand. Pain can produce sleep disturbance, immobility, lack of energy, and a reduced immune system, as well as provoke feelings of anger, anxiety, and fear. These symptoms and feelings are hard enough for an adult to endure, but they are almost impossible for a child to deal with or understand.

As discussed previously, stress in our society is rampant, sifting down to the adolescents and children. Many children and adolescents are devoid of a sense of

well-being. They are on medication, in therapy, and struggling socially and emotionally like no other generation before them. Migraine headaches in teenagers, as well as in children, are at an all-time high. Fibromyalgia, a debilitating disease with symptoms that include generalized, pain, muscle weakness, and depression, was once considered an adult ailment but now is fast becoming a pediatric diagnosis. Society at large must take a look at itself. We must recognize that these chronic, pain-ridden illnesses in children are a direct result of the ravages of stress in our children's lives.

stress related

Trauma is part of life, and accidents can happen. We can protect our children as much as possible with seatbelts, helmets, risk management, and safety knowledge, helping them to have an injury-free childhood. But we cannot protect them completely, so they could possiblty suffer a broken bone or laceration at any time. Pain from an injury is usually acute, but limited in its duration, such as when a child suffers from a fracture of the arm due to a fall from a bike. The acute injury of the broken bone and tissue damage are the primary sources of acute pain. Luckily, the bone can be put back together, and, with healing, the pain subsides and disappears. Imagery is useful in the control of acute pain whenever an injury occurs.

Chronic pain, on the other hand, is defined by pain that lasts more than three months. The cause is often unknown or unclear. A disease, a physical limitation, or a neurological impediment can produce this type of pain. The central nervous system carries pain signals to the brain, where they are given meaning. There are many causes for pain, both acute and chronic, and there are equally innumerable theories and research studies on the causes of pain. Put simply, pain is believed to be caused by a combination of neurological, muscular, and inflammatory events. But try explaining this to anyone in pain. When we're in pain, we don't really care where it comes from or how it all works. All we want is to get rid of it! This is where imagery as part of an overall wellness plan works wonders! With imagery, the cognitive support is in place, and with an established medical plan, the physical support is in place. The combination of the two creates a complementary power to heal and create wellness. This heightened power can overcome the power of pain.

Before doing this imagery exercise, ask your child to give you a number from one to ten, on a pain scale, with ten being the most severe pain and one being very mild pain. This will give you a benchmark to work with prior to doing the imagery. You can then check in after the relaxation piece and get another "reading" on the number the child allots to the pain. It can decrease a bit, just with the relaxation. At the end of the entire session, check the number again for the pain the child is experiencing. It has usually decreased, or is gone completely.

Do a relaxation exercise prior to this imagery.

You are taking quiet, deep breaths . . . relaxing your body . . . making yourself quiet and

calm ... letting go of any tension ... deeply
breathing ... listening to your breath ... starting
to decrease some of the body's tightness from
the pain.... Quietly and slowly, go to your special place ... and once you are there, relax and
take in all its peace and beauty ... slowly....
When you are ready, let an image of a measur-
ing device for your pain appear ... it can be anything ... a traffic light ... a thermometer ...
anything that can measure the pain you are feeling ... it can be anything at all. Just let it
form.... When the image comes to you, take
your time to look at it ... what do you see? ...
how does it work? ... ask it ... tell me more ...
let the image tell you how to use it ... it will
work. [Be patient and give time for the child to
do the work. Nothing should be rushed.] Let
the image help you decrease the pain you are
having right now ... [for example, it could be
numbered like a ruler, or color-related, such as
dark to light, etc.]. Now work with the measurement and decrease the number/color ...
[Encourage communication with the image.]
No rush ... let it happen ... staying relaxed ...
moving that number/color just a little ... you
can do it ... tell me more ... what is the number
now? ... Work with it some more ... decrease it

even more ... [Give time here and be patient.] You are feeling better ... more comfortable ... your pain has decreased ... perhaps it is even gone. Bring this feeling with you as far as you can today. When you are ready, begin to return to the room.... you are taking your time ... thinking of your breathing again ... hearing the sounds in the room ... slowly ... begin opening your eyes ... your body is relaxed, comfortable. It is nice to know that you are strong and able to help yourself whenever you need to.

Wrap-up: Ask questions: How do you feel? What do you think of the image that came to you? What does it mean? Can you continue to work with this image? Did your feelings change from the start of the session to the end of the session? Did you learn anything new today?

If the child is not your own, always get to know the person you are doing the imagery with first. I say this because I ran into a problem that I could have avoided if I had asked more in my initial intake of the patient during assessment. My patient was a fourteen-year-old girl with severe scoliosis, breathing problems, and multiple health issues. I was going to help her to relax, decrease her pain, and assist her to breathe more easily—or so I thought. I asked my standard questions

prior to the session, zeroing in on her health issues.
I thought I had collected enough information to begin
the imagery session. I was able to help her to relax
somewhat, though she could not perform any deep,
diaphragmatic breathing. She was reluctant to go to a
special place and was having difficulty imaging anything, which was out of the ordinary. When she did get
an image, it was of her grandmother's house, but she
began to appear somewhat ill at ease. We continued, and
I guided her to imagine her inner healer or advisor.
With some difficulty, she was able to image a fish in a
pond, briefly. But I could see she was becoming
intensely uncomfortable, moving around in her seat and
sadly starting to cry. Naturally I sensed that this experience was becoming a very negative, so we ended the session. In wrap-up she was quite sad and uncomfortable,
but she was unable to tell me why. We spent some time
discussing the imagery but gained no insight into the
problem. I felt I had not only not helped her, but I was
fearful that I had actually harmed her in some way.

Later I learned that she was a born-again Christian
and was absolutely horrified that I was guiding her into
using an image in nature and its creatures rather than a
spiritual figure, such as Jesus. She believed that all her
answers would come from Him and that it was wrong
to converse with a "fish" for assistance. It all fell into
place. I, unfortunately, had missed a key piece of information about her spiritual beliefs. If I had asked up
front about her beliefs, I could have honored them and
prepared to do the imagery in a way that would have

been comfortable for her, using symbols that embraced her faith. I now have on my patient information sheet a place where spiritual needs are addressed. And I always honor them, remembering that sad, distressed girl.

Evocative Imagery

ANOTHER POWERFUL TECHNIQUE in the imagery toolbag is evocative imagery. This involves recalling a time when a specific quality was in evidence—strength, for instance. Then, by the use of sensory recruitment, this experience is amplified and experienced again, subjectively. You as parent-guide help the child or teenager to summon this feeling or experience. Then, in times of illness (stress, etc.), the child can "get in touch" with this more positive quality once again. For example, I worked with a teenager who had lost the ability to participate in school sports (diving) due to fibromyalgia. With imagery, she could evoke a time of strength and grace experienced when she once performed the "perfect" dive during a past competition. Evoking this experience and feeling that strength, both physically and emotionally, was a positive experience in and of itself for her. But then she went on to apply it to the weakness and pain during fibromyalgia flare-ups, a practice that better enabled her to better control the symptoms. Thus she felt more empowered and positive. Such imaging is a powerful use of inner resources. If a child does not find the inner resources to draw upon, they can always use a hero figure or movie character to evoke certain strengths and qualities.

Do a relaxation exercise prior to this imagery.

Start to relax your body ... making yourself quiet and calm ... taking quiet, deep breaths ... letting go of any tension ... starting to decrease some of the tightness in the body ... deeply breathing ... listening to your breath ... aware of it and your body ... lightening ... when you are ready, let an image form. to represent this feeling or quality of [_____] that you experienced in the past ... [For a younger child, draw from a hero figure.] when you felt able, more in control of this feeling of [_____] ... take your time ... let it come ... it can be anything at all. Just let it form.... When this image comes, go to it, and imagine you are there.... [Be patient, and give time for the child to do the work. Nothing should be rushed.] Observe how it feels ... take in the different things about it.... Can you describe it? ... How do you feel? ... Where is it inside you? ... Tell me more ... [Encourage communication with the image.] Take your time, staying relaxed. (Going slowly, listening.) What does it look like? ... Now take that feeling of [_____], amplifying it, making it bigger ... feel it.... You can imagine actually turning up the volume on the quality or feeling.... Bring this feeling with you now. It is yours.... Now remember a problem or symptom that has troubled you....How does it feel?...Use this rediscovered feeling, and imagine dealing with whatever problem/symptom you have now.... What does it feel like?...Allow yourself to feel it...can it help you with your present concern or symptom? Stay with this feeling for a moment...enjoy it...you can have this feeling return whenever you want help. When you are ready, begin to return to the room...taking your time ... thinking of your breathing again ... hearing the sounds in the room ... slowly ... begin opening your eyes...your body is relaxed, comfortable. You can use this imagery anytime you wish.

Wrap-up: Ask questions: How do you feel? What were these images like? How did they make you feel? How do you feel about what happened? Can you work with these images again? Did your feelings change from the start of the session to the end of the session? Did you learn anything new today?

On rare occasions, a negative image can emerge. It may be an image that is frightening, sorrowful, or threatening. If this rarity should occur for your child or teen, you can handle it. Please note that imagery can be powerful. Staying with the process and trusting it are essential, making sure that the image is truly "bad." Sometimes it is simply the child or teen resisting a difficult feeling, a reluctannce to continue. Exploration of complex symptoms and feelings can cause fear and anxiety. You as the guide will have to decide if terminating the imagery is appropriate. Only mild anxiety should be accepted as okay. If you decide the child is having a negative experience and you are going to stop the imagery session, there are several things you can do. First, don't panic. Next, simply instruct the child to open the eyes slowly and return to the room, or tell the child to make the negative image go very far away and small. The child can also verbally banish the image or project themselves away from the image, leaving it far behind!

Glove Anesthesia
GLOVE ANESTHESIA is a fun and easy imagery technique to do. Kids especially like it. It is used primarily for the reduction of pain. The child simply uses imagery to make one hand numb or anesthetized, then places the numb hand on an area of pain. The imagery continues as the child imagines the area becoming numb, reducing the intensity of that area's pain. The parent is once again stimulating a sense, specifically the sense of touch.

The glove anesthesia technique works especially well with short-term pain from an injury, needle prick, or surgery. Nurses for post-operative patients have used this imagery technique in hospital settings, decreasing the use of pain medication. It also works well in a school setting. The child or teen can do it discreetly or in the nurse's office and return to class, rather than going home or taking medication.

Do a relaxation exercise prior to this imagery.

You are taking quiet, deep breaths ... relaxing your body ... making yourself quiet and calm ... letting go of any tension ... deeply breathing ... listening to your breath ... let an image form of a large bucket of numbing medicine (anesthetic). Go slowly ... there is no rush ... once you have that image, place one of your hands into the bucket ... feel the cold, numbing sensation ... swirl your hand around, noticing the feelings ... it is getting number and number ... cooler and cooler. Keep your hand in the solution as long as you can ... this feeling actually starts to go up your arm. ... When you are ready, take your numb, cool hand out of the bucket and place it on your [___]. Let the cold feeling spread into that area ... it is becoming numb too ... cooler ... and the pain is decreasing. The anesthetic is spreading. The pain is going away. You are feeling more comfortable and relaxed. Stay with this feeling. Know you can do this imagery anytime, anyplace, to help you with any discomfort you are having. Take this feeling with you as far as you can today. When you are ready, begin to return to the room . . . taking your time . . . thinking of your breathing again . . . hearing the sounds in the room . . . slowly . . . begin opening your eyes . . . your body is relaxed, comfortable. You can do this imagery anytime you need to.

Wrap-up: Ask questions: How do you feel? What was the use of that image like for you? What do you think of that image? Did your feelings change from the start of the session to the end of the session? Did you learn anything new today?

Conflict Resolution

ANOTHER METHOD the parent can use is imagery for conflict resolution. A good example (though not for children!) is that of the smoker. One part of that person wants to stop smoking, and the other, resistant, part wants to continue the behavior. This is a polarity—two parts on opposite ends of a continuum, often in conflict. In guided imagery, the child is guided to identify two (polar) inner aspects and then attempts to resolve the inner conflict, thus promoting wholeness by having these two images interact.

I worked with a nine-year-old child who was having trouble with her fourth-grade math. Her fear of math was becoming overwhelming and affecting the rest of her schoolwork. We tried imagery to resolve the conflict. Once she was relaxed and at her special place, she was asked to bring forward an image that represented her math. An image of a big, frowning "mean math face" came to her, and she looked obviously uncomfortable. Then she was asked to bring forward an image of her math the way she wanted it to be, which she described earlier as simply "easier." A large yellow "smiling good math face" came to her. She was then guided to have the two images speak to each other. (Remember, images can speak telepathically or verbally.) She explained that they were "arguing" about who was "right," when suddenly the image of the "mean face" started to get smaller. She then concentrated on that image exclusively, placing the "smiling face" to the side, and was able to diminish the "mean face" to a speck in the distance. She was literally smiling now and went back to the positive image, conversing with it and then thanking it.

When we discussed her imagery, she was very happy and felt she could do her math now because the bad math face had gone away. Now she was going to work with the smiling math face when she needed to, especially at school. Upon follow-up, she said she had worked with this image and her now-positive feelings toward math, and she had conquered her fear of math. Once that was done, she was able to go from a grade of D to a B in a short time!

Do a relaxation exercise prior to this imagery.

Relax with deep breaths ... once you are quiet, focused, and comfortable, let an image form of how you feel about [symptom or situation]. Take your time ... let it form on its own ... it will come ... there is no rush. (When you have the image, raise your finger or give a nod of your head.) Look at this image, and start to describe it ... how does it make you feel? ... Where does it occur in your body [if applicable]? Go slowly ... listen ... does this image have anything to say to you? What is it? Does this image have a name? If so, what is it? [Encourage communication with the image.] Once you have completed looking at this image, put it to the side for a moment. Now let an image form that is the opposite of [_____]or the positive of this situation or symptom. No rush ... let the image form on its own ... it can be anything at all ... just let it form. [Continue to communicate by a nod, etc.] Describe what it looks like. Be with the image, taking in the positive aspects of it. How does it feel? Where does it occur in your body? Does it have a name? Now, bring forward your previous image of [_____], and have the two images communicate with each other. What are

they saying? What is [____] (positive) saying?
What is [____] (negative) saying? [Be patient,
and give time for the child to do the work.
Nothing should be rushed.] Can they resolve
the problem? Do you have any questions to ask
[____]? Or [____]?

When you are ready, begin to return to the
room ... taking your time ... thinking of your
breathing again ... hearing the sounds in the
room ... slowly ... begin opening your eyes ...
your body is relaxed, comfortable.

Wrap up: Ask questions: How do you feel?
What do you think of these images? What was
using these images like for you? What do you
think these images mean? Did your feelings
change from the start of the session to the end of
the session? Did you learn anything new today?

Transforming Pain

THIS IMAGERY is unique because you work with the
combination of imagery and drawing. I have found it
extremely useful when working with children and adolescents. It is a way for the child or teen to modulate the
pain and is empowering over the symptoms. The child
draws on a body diagram (see the figures on the following page) where the pain is. This first drawing is the
pain at its "worst," the second drawing is the pain at its

"best," and the third drawing depicts the pain when it is gone. Ask the child or teen to draw these three representations of the pain prior to the imagery session itself. Let the child take some time to depict every detail. You need three diagrams and colored crayons or pencils. Prior to doing relaxation and the imagery, discuss the drawings, and make notes on anything significant the child says about the drawings and any feelings about them. Next, explain that, during the

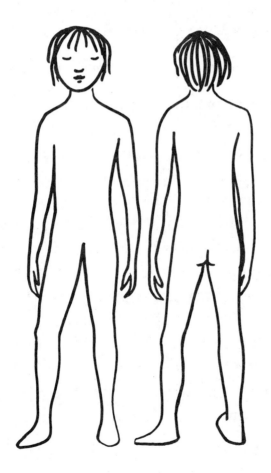

imagery, the drawings will be used again to change or transform the pain and that the primary outcome is to be as pain free as possible. With imagery the child can picture the pain at its worst, like the drawing, and then move down the path to the next drawing, and subsequently decrease the pain level. After working with the second drawing, the child can move along the path again to the picture that is pain free. Think of this imagery technique as a map of a three-step path that the child has drawn. The child can follow this path while relaxed and doing the imagery.

Do a relaxation excercise prior to this imagery.

Relax and breathe deeply.... Once you are quiet, focused, and comfortable, let the picture of your first drawing come to you. Take your time ... staying relaxed ... focused ... when you see it, let me know.... Describe the first drawing of your pain ... how does it make you feel inside? ... Has the drawing changed in any way? ... Tell me more.... When you are ready, bring forward your second drawing ... again taking your time. Can you describe it to me? ... How does this picture feel to you? ... Tell me more ... [Encourage interaction with the image.] What is your pain like now? ... Has the drawing changed in any way? ... When you are ready, go on to your last drawing ... What do you see?

How does this last drawing make you feel? ... Describe it. ... How is your pain now? ... Go on. Stay with this last image, and bring its feeling of decreased pain (or no pain) as far into your day as possible.

Wrap-up: Ask questions: How do you feel? What was using these drawings like for you? Do you think you could use this imagery again? Were you able to decrease your pain? How did it feel when your drawings changed (if applicable)? Did your feelings change from the start of the session to the end of the session? Did you learn anything new today?

Color is an important aspect of this imagery as is its place in the body. I am not a professional color therapist, but I did do some research on the significance of color. The following is a brief overview. White has the quality of all colors and has a healing aspect to it. Purple is inspirational, represents sensitivity and spirituality, a mix of blue (knowledge) and red (activity). Blue indicates peace, truth, health, and knowledge. Green is the color of balance, self-control, endurance, and growth. Yellow signifies warmth, spontaneity, cheer, radiance, and clarity. Orange is creativity and energy. Red is also energy, as well as vitality, self-confidence, and passion. This information about color is just another tool for

your imagery toolbag, a tool that can bring further insight to the experience, for both your child and you. Of course, there are many books on this subject that are extremely interesting if you require further details on the meaning of color.

Six: The World of Teenagers

"WE KNOW WHAT WE ARE BUT KNOW NOT WHAT WE MAY BE."

-Anonymous

THE WORD TEENAGER does not mean what it used to mean. In our fast-forward society, adolescence now begins in the eight- to ten-year-old age group. The children of the world are growing up much earlier than they were even a decade ago. The "tweens," as they have been dubbed by marketers, are not playing with dolls and trucks but trying to score rock concert tickets. They are defined as the twenty-seven million children between the ages of eight and twelve, the baby-sized version of a teenager. Many of them dress older (demanding designer labels) and, therefore, look older, but their maturity is not in place. This conflict causes an array of problems. Tweens are consumers before their time. These kids find themselves in the confusing state of not being a child anymore but not yet being a teen. There are many reasons for this—today's marketing, movies, TV, single-parent families, kids shouldering more responsibility, and the Internet, to name just a few. It boils down to the sheer exposure these children have. Developmentally, they are forming a sense of self, but social acceptance is of most importance. Normal neurological and social growth are at their peaks. This is a time of friendships, passwords, rituals, and bonding. Friends are usually of the same sex, but interest in the opposite sex is increasing. There are also bodily changes, which can be confusing enough. Schoolwork becomes more demanding, peer pressure increases on a daily basis, and competition in sports and academics rises. For children, stress issues, behavioral problems, and illnesses are the negative spin-off from our hyperactive society.

Many of the issues faced by these prepubescents have come directly from the situation of "growing up" that teenagers have always endured. The teenagers of the new millennium have been seriously affected by today's stresses. They not only have concerns about body image, peer acceptance, and dating but also must endure extreme forms of competition regarding school, money, and social prowess. Puberty is well under way, rules are being tested, and autonomy is struggling to evolve. It is well known that teenagers often become challenging and opinionated, often causing conflict at home and at school. Teenagers are learning to drive, usually working a job, and often starting to have relationships with the opposite sex. Risk-taking behavior can emerge in the form of experimentation with alcohol, drugs, and sex. It can be a time of moods, feelings of sadness, disappointments, and losses.

With all this in mind, imagine the child or teen who may already have a health issue such as asthma, chronic pain, or diabetes. These children have endured a lot and, thus, can draw on an inner strength that comes from a sense of how recognizing their illness affects them. They also can have a fragile side which is intolerant of daily pressures and expectations. This kind of child or adolescent has to walk a fine line between feeling "different" and needing to be accepted. This delicate situation is just as difficult for the parent to understand and support. The restrictions imposed on a chronically ill or temporarily ill child or teen can make it hard to gain acceptance by peers. When a child is struggling with a health issue, activities such as sports must often be abandoned or reduced, making their young lives even more stressful. Physical strength and emotional well-being are not guaranteed during the course of a chronic illness. The situation can be unpredictable, increasing fear, frustration, and anxiety for the child. Even a short-term illness or injury can affect a teen's life negatively, like missing the championship game or the prom. Generally a sick child can become resentful of an illness, and become uncooperative. The child, especially a teen, can become noncompliant, refusing treatments or medications. The parent then has the important job of preventing the child or adolescent from becoming more ill or incapacitated. This can be a real challenge. Ask any parent of a diabetic teenager.

Some basic goals for the parent of an adolescent with an illness are to keep communication open, to discuss treatment plans, to give options, to monitor school activities and attendance, to allow some autonomous problem-solving, and to keep illness separate from social issues.

I have found that adolescents enjoy imagery. They may not show the enthusiasm of younger children, but it comes through in other ways—a quick smile, a relaxed, quiet body, or tears of relief. It is a challenge to get them to listen to how the process works—talk about skeptics! But as they nonchalantly ignore some of my introduction, I always know they are hearing some of it too. I like to let them know that imagery is like going to the movies, but it is their movie!

I do a relaxation and a special place imagery to start. I watch body language closely. Teenagers are extremely self-conscious, so I try to make the setting comfortable, quiet, and as nonthreatening as possible. You might want to pick an area in your home that will create this kind of feeling. I ask them to pick out music they might want to listen to, giving them only two or three choices, such as Native American or Asian music. Then I just go for it. In my entire practice, I have had to end only two sessions with teenagers. One was due to increased discomfort (see pg. 124), and the other was because of noncompliance. When a child is just not going to do it, I do not want to waste my time or the family's time. Often the first session is difficult, and I get the feeling the teen got absolutely nothing out of it. The imagery is bland, the images do not communicate, and there is no focus, no relaxation. Then the teenager claims to have learned "nothing" from the session in the end. The surprise here is that these teens come back. They go home, and the imagery process continues. They get to the privacy of their own rooms and then do the imagery for themselves—many times creating magnificent images that really have an impact on their symptoms. When they come for their second session, I find this out. I also see a different type of attitude, more of a kinship with me as a practitioner, and a belief in the imagery process itself. They carry a newfound knowledge, which I can hear without them saying anything. There is eye contact and a smile of gratitude that is hard to miss. They have learned to trust the process. As they say, it can be cool.

Guided Imagery for Teens

"IMAGERY IS THE LANGUAGE OF THE MIND."
                                    —Dr. Martin Rossman

The Beauty in You (Body Image)

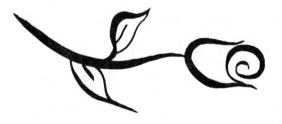

This imagery can be used for body image.
Do a relaxation exercise prior to this imagery.

ONCE you have done your relaxation and you are ready and comfortable, let an image form of your special place. Get comfortable in your special place, and then let an image appear of yourself. Take your time. Open up to the small quiet voice within. Look at yourself, and begin to observe the good things about your body. Go inside, and use new eyes to see it, understanding and appreciating that you have not seen your body in this clear light before. Notice that you are graceful, strong, and light. You have never felt such lightness. Look more closely, and see your inner strength and grace. Take your time. There is no rush. Step into this image of yourself . . . making it fit, making it real. Feel how good you feel in your body. No other body is better for you. If your critical mind enters this place, send it away. There is no negative energy toward you here. There is no inner critic here, only self-love and beauty. Stand in your special place, and observe yourself from all angles slowly, inside and outside. Let yourself watch the lengthening and lightening of your body, mind, and spirit. You are able to see the small, subtle changes your body is having, today. Let them happen, just go with it. You are flexible, strong, and happy. Trust the process, and let it happen. Give time to continue to observe the image. Stay as long as you like, feeling this new freedom in body as well as mind. Enjoy your inner beauty, your inner strength and power. When it is time, start to walk away from your special, safe place, saying good-bye and thank you. You are filled with appreciation and happiness. With each step, you become lighter, more agile, smoother. Be mindful that, with each step you take, there is a small change occurring, your body changing, becoming whatever you need to become. Your inner splendor and gracefulness are alive and real, today. As your image fades, stay relaxed and comfortable. Hold onto the lightness and strength that you have found today, and bring it with you as far into your day as possible. You are feeling refreshed and revitalized.

Recall: Anytime you wish, you can softly close your eyes, return to your special place, and see yourself once again as light and graceful, full of beauty, strength, and happiness, stepping lightly and softly. And you enjoy being in your body, your form. Light, free, powerful, and loved.

The Silver Forest (Wound Healing)

This imagery can be used for wound healing.
Do a relaxation exercise prior to this imagery.

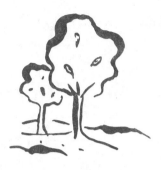

Once you are comfortable and relaxed, imagine walking through the thick lush carpet of green meadow grass. You are barefoot and the grass feels cool and soft under your feet. It smells like a mixture of wind, clover, and sunshine, and it's the sweetest smell you have ever experienced. As you walk, you hear the light song of the birds in the air overhead and feel the warm, pure wind run its fingers over your face. You are feeling happy and safe, though your wound [laceration, broken bone] is bothering you a bit. Somewhere deep inside, though, you know this is a healing place. Just ahead of you is a beautiful, emerald-green hill with a grove of shimmering, silver trees on its crest. You have never seen anything like these trees before. Their leaves are cut crystal and catch the light like little prisms, sending off millions of tiny rainbows. The trunks of these trees are twisted silver and gold, sparkling, and strong. As you walk toward the hill and

Teens

begin to climb its slow slope, you realize that you are here for a reason. You are here to heal your wound (laceration, broken bone). This is a magical place with awesome power. Your eyes are fixed on the magnificent trees as you walk toward them. You cannot take your eyes off them. You come to the first tree and lay your hand slowly on one of its iridescent branches, and you immediately feel stronger. You rest your forehead on its golden, silvery bark, and it cools and refreshes you. You lose track of time ... resting, quiet, leaning on this powerful, splendid tree. Slowly you notice the sound of soft, whispered singing. It is magical. You turn and walk into the grove of silver trees and stand in the center, the prismed light and fantastic song surrounding you. The soft grass under your feet beckons you to lie down in it. You relax and stretch out in the tender, sweet, and shimmering grass. The crystal leaves turn inward to you. The sunlight reflects through them, and all their powerful rainbowed light is focused on the pain in your [_____]. Let this powerful, colored light take your pain away. It fills your skin, your bones, with its color and warmth. You can feel it healing your [_____]. You have no pain, and you feel strong. [Go slowly. Give time to the child.]

Stay and listen to the music and feel this comfortable feeling as long as you like, your body and mind drinking in this healing from the silver forest. This is your special place, here for you whenever you need it.

Recall: Anytime you wish, you can softly close your eyes and return to your silver forest. Relax and breathe deeply, and see yourself once again walking toward the hill and its magnificent crown of silver and gold trees. You can see the prisms sparkling from the leaves, and you know how that will feel when you get there. You know it will help your discomfort and make you strong and happy. Go there whenever you want ...it's here for you.

The Trekking Dial
PEGASUS (DIFFICULTY BREATHING)

This imagery can be used for difficulty breathing.
Do a relaxation exercise prior to this imagery.

YOU are starting to have some trouble breathing, and you need your medicine. Take it, and start to relax your body. Once you have done your relaxation and you are ready, you can help yourself to feel better and more in control.

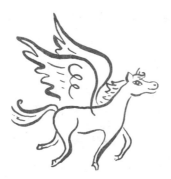

While you quiet yourself, imagine a beautifully carved wooden chest with a hinged top. Its surfaces are covered with images of faraway places and incredible creatures. While your medication starts to work, somehow you realize that the chest contains something else that can also help you breathe better, something really different. You quickly and easily raise its heavy cover, and, inside, you discover a large brass dial. You lift the dial out of the chest. It has the same incredible pictures the chest has. There is a handle in the middle of the dial. On it are the words in fancy letters: "The Trekking Dial." You can turn it to any picture you want.... The horse with wings looks interesting. There is also something else written there: "A winged steed, unwearying of flight, sweeping through air, swift as a gale of wind." You point the dial to its picture.

Suddenly you are flying through the brilliant, blue sky, with the rush of cool, clean air all around you! Your lungs are opening and filling with this wonderful, healing air, and you can breathe. A solid, white cloud-cover carpets the sky below, and you feel totally fearless.

At first you are surprised, but within seconds you realize that you are not alone. Your hands tightly clutch the coarse hair of a golden mane; your legs feel the movement of the powerful chest as the extraordinary, flying horse breathes and snorts boldly through the sky. You can feel his great heartbeat, and it feels like your own, as if together you are all one being. This is Pegasus, from ancient Greek mythology, who has come to help you. Pegasus, the lord of the air, has tremendously strong wings that can take you anywhere. You can feel the rhythm of his great wings as they move you both through the heavens. He will bring you aloft into the endless sky, where the rushing winds help you to stop wheezing and coughing. Your hand touches his mighty, winged shoulder. You have never felt such strength in your life. You feel strong, unafraid, and happy. You can breathe without any trouble with the power of Pegasus. All the air around you is healing. Each breath you take fills your lungs to capacity, unblocking the tubes and opening all your airways—even the tiny ones. He has done his job; you are breathing with no trouble.

You want to go on forever, flying with Pegasus. But you realize you must go home for now, and he must return to his magical place.

He breaks through the cloud-cover and you see the world for an instant . . . and then it is gone. You are back, relaxed, strong, comfortable, quietly breathing. You feel safe, yet tingling all over because of the thrill you have just had. You realize that with the fantastic Trekking Dial you can travel anywhere with anyone, and clear your lungs at the same time!

Recall: You can use your Trekking Dial anytime you wish, especially if you are having any trouble breathing. It is for you and you alone. You can bring Pegasus back anytime, anyplace, and take your amazing ride. Just relax and deeply breathe. Go to the dial and imagine turning it to your famous horse. You know he can help you. You can clear and open your lungs to the fresh, brisk air that comes when you ride him. You can ride him anytime you wish!

The Oxygen Planet (Asthma Symptoms)

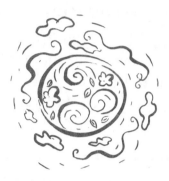

This imagery can be used for asthma symptoms.
Do a relaxation exercise prior to this imagery.

Once you have done your relaxation and you are ready, you can help yourself feel better. Whenever you start to have trouble breathing—with wheezing, coughing, and chest tightness—you can go to your mystical chest and get your brass Trekking Dial. This fantastic dial can take you anywhere. Your choices are limitless, so after you take your medication, relax your body and try to slow your breathing. The dial has so many pictures to choose from. This time you turn the knob to a picture of a mysterious planet. It reads, "The story of man's greatest feat of exploration."

At once, you are travelling faster than the speed of light into the vast openness of space. You are protected by a powerful force field, and somehow you are travelling without the aid of a spacecraft. The power comes from within you. Your mission is to reach the magnificent planet ahead of you. You can think of nothing else or see nothing else ... just your powerful planet.

In a flash you are there, breathing the sweetest, purest air you have ever encountered. This planet is the oxygen planet. It is healing to your lungs. It is the best place in the galaxy for you to be. Your lungs are responding immediately, and you can breathe without effort. You feel weightless, calm, and absolutely unafraid. This is your special place, so name the planet any name you want.

You feel so good, and breathing is so easy that you start to explore, forgetting why you came here in the first place. You're no longer worrying about an asthma attack!

As you look around, you see the most incredible sights; there are large craters in the distance that look iridescent in the reflection of the sun's light. There are three moons in the sky, strange and beautiful. You see magnificent mountains of crystal rock with rainbow-colored waterfalls. There are limitless valleys of some kind of plant that pumps pure oxygen into the atmosphere continuously. No wonder this is the perfect place for you! Your lungs feel brand-new, healthy, and perfect. You could explore and live here forever . . . but you realize you need to get home. Before you go, take with you this feeling of perfect and strong lungs, and keep it with you. You know you can come back anytime.

You launch off the planet's surface as fast as when you left Earth. You hurl toward Earth and home, again arriving, incredibly, within seconds. You stand in front of the carved chest with the Trekking Dial in your hands. Your breathing is calm and soft, controlled. You put your dial away for now. knowing you can travel to your planet anytime, anyplace.

Recall: Anytime you wish, bring out your Trekking Dial and travel to your planet. It can help you whenever you need it to, especially when you have trouble breathing. Relax and go, clear and open your lungs. It is your special planet, and it's for you alone. Enjoy the freedom, the extraordinary landscapes, and your quiet, easy, healed breathing.

In the Canopy (General)

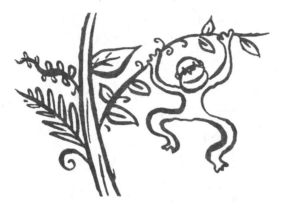

This imagery can be used for generalized symptoms.
Do a relaxation exercise prior to this imagery.

ONCE you have done your relaxation and you are ready, go to your Trekking Dial. The Trekking Dial has given you a way to control what happens to you when you are sick. The dial makes it possible for you go to a new place, and meet new people and creatures, whenever you want. It is an incredible and fantastic tool for you to have, and you can use it whenever your symptoms flare up.

As you sit holding the Trekking Dial in your lap, you are studying its many pictures of far-away places and things. You have always wondered about one of its pictures. It looks like a sky full of trees. You are curious to see what this place is. You point to the intriguing picture that says, "Save the Rainforest."... Instantly the air is warm and humid, and you hear the sounds of a dense jungle. The warmth fills your body, replacing that sick and uncomfortable feeling the illness gave you. You feel this warmth immediately and become less tense, your body more relaxed. You relax enough to hear monkeys chattering, birds calling, and the strange humming and whirling of insects. You feel light and aloft. You get your bearings and see you are actually in the rainforest, way high up in its canopy. The air you breathe is almost pure oxygen, produced from the mighty jungle trees. Each breath you take alleviates your symptoms. You are on a perch at the top of the highest tree in all the land, enabling you to see for miles across the top layer of the canopy. You have absolutely no fear. Activists who want to save the rainforest have built this platform at the top of the tree, where they live so it cannot be cut down; this "tree perching" saves the life of the tree. A very clever idea, indeed. Now you are there, in this unique place, getting the personal benefit of the purest air on the earth. Your breathing is perfect and easy. Your pain, sick feeling, and any other symptoms are decreasing quickly. This is an extraordinary place that not many human beings get to see. You are one of the fortunate ones, looking out over some of the most lush, untouched land on the planet. How lucky you are! How powerful—you can accomplish anything here. Most of all, you can overcome your symptoms. Relax, sleep if you want, and rid your body of all tension and discomfort.

When you are ready, you need to return home. But remember this healing place, and bring it back with you in your heart. Bring your quiet, happy, strong body with you as far as you can today.

Recall: You can come here any time, whenever you need to clear your lungs, or to be alone, or to gain your strength. You can decrease any symptoms you may be having. Just relax and breathe deeply, and turn the dial to return to your perch. This position of extraordinary strength protects you from the pain. Use it wherever you want, anytime.

The Tapestry Shawl (Inner Strength)

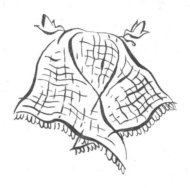

This imagery can be used for coping/inner strength.
Do a relaxation exercise prior to this imagery.

ONCE you are relaxed and deeply comfortable, imagine a lush meadow with a shimmering river running through it. Beyond the river is a cool, deep wood. You can hear the soft, light sounds of the river splashing over and around its stone floor. There is a warm breeze. It brings protection and calm. This breeze carries with it the sounds of the woods and the smell of rich, clean water. Every breath you take fills you with quiet serenity, opening you up to the small quiet voice within. You begin to walk slowly, through the meadow, toward the river. With each step, you shed all your burdens, all your worries and sorrows. You are alone, feeling light and strong. You are lifted as you walk.

At the river's edge stands a large, wooden loom and a woven basket full of extraordinary yarns. These yarns are of every color imaginable. And you want to touch them. So your walk quickens, anticipating their sumptuous textures.

You reach the loom, sitting down to its perfect fit. Your hands touch the magnificent yarn. You caress and lift its luxurious softness to your face. You breathe in its warm lanolin smell. This yarn gives you knowledge and strength, and you are well and powerful.

You set to work at the loom, feeding it strands of yarn, nourishing it. The act of weaving nourishes you, as well. The smooth sound of wood against wood hums from the loom each time you add a color and tighten the weave. Without putting any thought to it, slowly a magnificent pattern appears. The rich purples and strong hues of greens and blues dazzle you. There are endless colors for you to use. Your mixture of colors is indescribable, and your soft fabric is sturdy. You have done a good job. You carefully and lovingly remove your tapestry from the loom. You wrap it around your shoulders, and it covers your entire back and your arms. It is your tapestry shawl, a shield to use whenever you need its comfort and protection. The power it holds for you is simple: it can give you the gift of "peace of mind." A restful, quiet self. A strong and unyielding inner spirit. An ability to be in a quiet, silent place, without fear. You created it. And you can create healing and happiness in your life.

Recall: Whenever you need your tapestry shawl, you can easily bring it out whenever you want. Do your relaxation exercise. When you are relaxed and ready, return to the green meadow and sparkling river. Imagine your loom, and set to work making your beautiful tapestry. Wrap yourself in the marvelous material and feel its power. It is your shield, to help and protect you. You can have your shawl anytime, anyplace.

The Big White House (Stress/Burdens)

This imagery can be used to decrease stress.
Do a relaxation exercise prior to this imagery.

IMAGINE walking along a long white beach. You can hear the gulls and the gentle roll of the

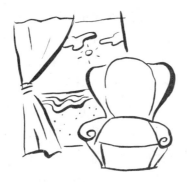

waves. Your feet sink into the warm, white sand. It is quiet and safe. You are alone walking into the soft sea wind. The sun is shining down on you, making you warm. You have been looking for a place to be quiet and comfortable. This feels as if it is your beach, yours alone. You stop and stand, looking out over the immense, expanding ocean. It shows its green top-water, its purple mid-water, and its gray powerful underwater. The colors are mixing and churning, creating the bubbly white crest at the top of each wave. The roll of each wave sounds like the Earth, breathing. O . . . cean. O . . . cean. Over and over again with each wave. You feel the power of the ocean and the Earth. A short distance ahead of you, you now notice a big, white house. It is beckoning to you. It looks like a temple or small castle of some sort. You walk toward it, relaxed and interested. You follow a

short path to the house and see that the large
door is open. You feel that it perfectly okay for
you to go inside. It is safe and calm. You step
out of the sunshine and into the coolness of this
beautiful house. You find yourself in a huge
hallway with plants and paintings. A magnificent, marble staircase stands before you. You
know you want to go up those stairs. You
become aware of a very heavy backpack that
you have been carrying all this time. The backpack is full of your worries, troubles, concerns,
and negative feelings. You have been carrying
them for a long time, and you realize that this
backpack is weighting you down. Your shoulders ache, and your back feels tight and stiff
from all these feelings. Slowly remove your
backpack and, with it, all your worries and concerns. You feel released, free! You can now easily ascend the staircase. Each step you take, you
become lighter, happier, and quieted. Each step
brings you closer to absolute comfort and joy.
The comfort and joy live in you, and now there
is nothing to get in the way of feeling them,
reaching them, having comfort and joy. Now at
the top of the stairs, you are strong and certain.
A large window is open at the top of the stairs,
and in front of it is a big, white comfortable

chair. You sit down and face the window, watching the magnificent ocean once again. This time is yours. You watch from your chair, by your window in your house. Breathe in the soft ocean air, and know you are home.

Recall: You can come here any time, whenever you need to relax and quiet yourself. Deeply breathe and relax, and settle into yourself. Imagine walking on your beach, to your house. Remember to leave your backpack at the bottom of the stairs. Leave your burdens and worries behind.

Teens

Conclusion

The Unbreakable Bond

"THE SOUL IS HEALED BY BEING WITH CHILDREN."
-Fyodor Dostoyevski

You now have many techniques to choose from in using imagery. I hope that you are feeling more in tune with the process as a whole and that you feel as if you can guide with comfort and confidence your child or teen. As you now know, imagery does not stop when the session stops. It is an ongoing experience, bringing your child or teen new feelings and insights over time. You may wonder, what is the next step for your parent-child team? What do you do with this information, and how do you assist your child further? The next step is to simply trust the process, and your child. You have become the guardian of extraordinary knowledge, which brings to your loved ones (and to yourself) well-being, vitality, inner strength, and endurance—through self-healing.

For our family, the Blue Whales, and imagery as a whole, have become an intricate part of our daily lives. Allison and I are involved intimately with the Blue Whale imagery and with all kinds of healing imagery as mother and daughter, as well as nurse and patient. The special bond that was created by our collaboration in the imagery process is one that is unshakable, filled with deep trust and love. I believe it can never be broken. I share this bond with my other growing daughter as well.

Writing this book was the path I chose in order to work through my fear and anger about my daughter's illness. This creative process has brought me to a place of strength, acceptance, and peace. As mother and daughter, we have created a way to work together to counteract the disease process. This experience has shaped and changed our lives in many positive, wondrous ways. Most importantly, Allison is well.

For me, I have gone on to become certified in Interactive Guided Imagery^{SM} and have a private practice specializing in imagery for healing children. I have developed a workshop for children and their parents, which includes yoga and guided imagery. Sharing this unique technique in imagery is our way of spreading the joy of self-healing to others in need. Using imagery is an enriching and empowering experience for you and your loved ones. Trust the process. It opens the creative and healing spirit that lives within us all.

Professional Training Resources

For more information on guided imagery training, please contact:

Nurses' Certificate Program in Imagery
Beyond Ordinary Nursing
P.O. Box 8177
Foster City, CA 94404
(650) 570-6157
NCPII@aol.com
http://www.imageryrn.com

Academy for Guided Imagery
P.O. Box 2070
Mill Valley, CA 94942
(800) 726-2070 or (415) 389-9325
AGI1996@aol.com
http://www.interactiveimagery.com

Notes

1. Herbert Benson and Marg Stark, *Timeless Healing* (New York: Scribner, 1996), 144.

2. Herbert Benson and William Proctor, *Beyond the Relaxation Response* (New York: Time Books, 1984), 47-50.

3. Andrew Weil, "The Power of Guided Imagery," *Self Healing* (2000).

4. Alice Domar and Henry Dreher, "New Research" http://www.healthjourneys.com.

5. Benson, *Beyond the Relaxation Response*, 5.

6. "Journal Writing," *New Age* (Nov. 1999): 58.

7. http://www.interactiveimagery.com

8. The Burton Goldberg Group, *Alternative Medicine: The Definitive Guide* (Puyallap, Wash.: Future Medicine Publishing, 1994), 346-48.

Bibliography

Benson, Herbert, *The Relaxation Response.* (New York: Murrow, 1975).

Benson, Herbert, Eileen Stuart, and the staff of the Mind/Body Institute, *The Wellness Book* (New York: Fireside, 1993).

Caudill, Margaret, *Managing Pain before It Manages You* (New York: Guilford Press, 1995).

Jahnke, Roger, *The Healer Within* (San Francisco: HarperCollins Publishing, 1999).

Moynihan, Patricia M., and Broatch Haig, *Whole Parent Whole Child* (Minnnesota: DCI Publishing, 1989).

Naparstek, Belleruth, *Staying Well with Guided Imagery* (New York: Warner Books, 1995).

Rossman, Martin, *Guided Imagery for Self-Healing: An Essential Resource for Anyone Seeking Wellness* (California: HJ Kramer, 2000).

Shames, Karilee Halo, *Creative Imagery in Nursing* (New York: Delmar Publishing, 1995).

"Stress," *Newsweek* (June 1999): 56.

"Tweens," *Newsweek* (Oct. 1999): 62.

Weil, Andrew, *Spontaneous Healing* (New York: Ballantine Books, 1995).

http://www.imageryrn.com

http://www.kidshealth.org

http://www.pathfinder.com/drwiel

Raising Children Who Think for Themselves
Author: Elisa Medhus, M.D.
$14.95, softcover

Raising Children Who Think for Themselves offers a new approach to parenting that has the power to reverse the trend of external direction in children—that tendency to make decisions based on outside influences—and help parents bring up empathetic, self-confident, moral, independent thinkers. Filled with real-life examples, humorous anecdotes, and countless interviews with parents, children, and teachers, this book identifies the five essential qualities of self-directed children, outlines the seven strategies necessary for parents to develop these qualities in their children, and offers solutions to nearly one hundred child-raising challenges.

Nurturing Your Child with Music
How Sound Awareness Creates Happy, Smart, and Confident Children
Author: John M. Ortiz, Ph.D.
$14.95, softcover

Author and psychomusicologist Dr. John Ortiz says that we have "just begun to tap into the powers behind the timeless element of sound," and in his book *Nurturing Your Child with Music*, Dr. Ortiz allows the readerss to discover those musical powers through and with their children. Designed for parents who take an active interest in their children's lives, this book offers a number of creative methods through which families can initiate, enhance, and maintain happy, relaxed, and productive home environments. *Nurturing Your Child with Music* includes easy-to-do exercises and fun activities to bring music and sound into parenting styles and family life. The book provides music menus and sample "days of sound" to use during the prenatal, newborn, preschool, and school-age phases. Dr. Ortiz shares how we can keep our family "in tune" and create harmony in our homes by inviting music and sound into our daily dance of life.

A Guy's Guide to Pregnancy:
Preparing for Parenthood Together
Author: Frank Mungeam; Foreword: John Gray, Ph.D.
$12.95, softcover

Every day, four thousand American men become first-time dads. There are literally hundreds of pregnancy guidebooks aimed at women, but guys rarely rate more than a footnote. *A Guy's Guide to Pregnancy* is the first book to explain in "guy terms" the changes that happen to a man's partner and their relationship during pregnancy, using a humorous yet insightful approach. Future fathers will find out what to expect when they enter the "Pregnancy Zone." *A Guy's Guide to Pregnancy* is designed to be guy-friendly—approachable in appearance as well as content and length. It is divided into forty brisk chapters, one for each week of the pregnancy.

Nurturing Spirituality in Children
Author: Peggy J. Jenkins, Ph.D.
$10.95, softcover

Children who develop a healthy balance of mind and spirit enter adulthood with high self-esteem, better able to respond to life's challenges. Many parents wish to heighten their children's spiritual awareness but have been unable to find good resources. *Nurturing Spirituality in Children* offers scores of simple lessons that parents can teach to their children in less than ten minutes at a time.

Discovering Another Way

Raising Brighter Children While Having a Meaningful Career
Author: Lane Nemeth
$16.95, softcover

Discovery Toys is a pioneer in the educational toy market. *In Discovering Another Way*, founder Lane Nemeth tells how she built this $100 million company from the ground up, a company that helped change the lives of tens of thousands of women and an entire generation of kids who have grown up smarter in "Discovery Toys Families." The book provides a refreshingly candid insider's view of how to start your own business *and* follow your heart, enriching your children's minds and imaginations *at the same time*. It is also a heartwarming story of Lane Nemeth's dedication to bring quality toys that spark a sense of discovery and learning to all children, not just a chosen few. Interspersed throughout Lane's story are chapters revealing the gems of parenting wisdom she discovered while raising her family and her business: "So You Want a Cooperative Child?," "Guidelines for Brain-Building Play," "How to Turn Your Child into a Lifelong Reader," and "Five Ways to Enhance Your Time with Your Child." Lane explains the magic of learning moments and shows parents how to turn every occasion into an opportunity for discovery and learning.

To order or request a catalog, contact
Beyond Words Publishing, Inc.
20827 N.W. Cornell Road, Suite 500
Hillsboro, OR 97124-9808
503-531-8700 or 1-800-284-9673

You can also visit our Web site at *www.beyondword.com* or e-mail us at *info@beyondword.com.*

Beyond Words Publising, Inc.

Our corporate mission:

Inspire to Integrity

Our declared values:

We give to all of life as life has given us.
We honor all relationships.
Trust and stewardship are integral to fulfilling dreams.
Collaboration is essential to create miracles.
Creativity and aesthetics nourish the soul.
Unlimited thinking is fundamental.
Living your passion is vital.
Joy and humor open our hearts to growth.
It is important to remind ourselves of love.